THE SEVEN KEYS TO
COLOR HEALING

P9-BJR-761

THE SEVEN KEYS
TO
COLOR HEALING

Diagnosis and Treatment Using Color

Roland Hunt, A.M.I.C.A., Ms.D., Ps.D.

With a foreword by
Ivah B. Whitten, A.M.I.C.A.

1817

HARPER & ROW, PUBLISHERS, San Francisco
Cambridge, Hagerstown, New York, Philadelphia
London, Mexico City, São Paulo, Sydney

THE SEVEN KEYS TO COLOR HEALING
Diagnosis and Treatment Using Color

First Harper & Row paperback edition published in 1982.

Library of Congress Cataloging in Publication Data

Hunt, Roland T.
   The seven keys to color healing.

   (Harper library of spiritual wisdom)
   Bibliography: p. 121
   Includes index.
   1. Color—Therapeutic use. I. Title. II. Series:
Harper's library of spiritual wisdom.
RM840.H86   615.8'31   81-47849
ISBN 0-06-064080-4   AACR2

83 84 85 86   10 9 8 7 6 5 4 3

THE SEVEN KEYS TO
COLOR HEALING

In the beginning of this epoch was given to the World the Rainbow symbol of Great Promise: "I do set My *bow* in the cloud, and it shall be for a token of a covenant between Me and the Earth" (Genesis).

Again, at the end of the Rainbow, Man has ever sought the legendary "Pot of Gold" to bring him Happiness.

Now, out of the cloud of dark ages, Science and Philosophy agree with the promise of Ancient Wisdom and legend alike, that the Rainbow's promise and treasure lie not in the earth but in the skies of *Consciousness*.

DEDICATED
TO MY MOTHER

CONTENTS

7

FOREWORD

THE manuscript of this book comes into my hands at a time when gallant England is crucially involved in a fight for life, and indeed, civilization as we know it, when so much chaos and destruction have been loosed upon the world by the forces of darkness.

In these circumstances, and with all the attendant difficulties conspiring to upset the normal rhythm in writing and publishing, it is remarkable and utterly praiseworthy that such a splendid constructive healing effort, carrying the torch of Light and Colour, should be put forward to relieve and raise stricken humanity.

I therefore extend to Mr. Hunt and his publishers my admiration for their courage and resourcefulness in presenting this timely and urgently needed work to "fill the breach" for "Using Colour." I can but add—"that which is done in times of stress is doubly done!"

Colour-breathing, mentioned for the first time in this book as an integral part of the prescribed Colour-treatments, is in fact the greatest of all advanced methods and is destined to restore the coming New Race to its God-given physical perfection.

Thus you may judge for yourself just how valuable this book is destined to become to the world, holding as it does the *key* to colour-breathing together with sane, easily understood instructions leading up to this end.

Roland Hunt has the happy faculty of rationalizing the teachings he passes on to his reading public, marking the path his writings indicate in simple, understandable fashion.

You are, to-day, the product of your Colour responses to the various circumstances through which you have passed, during the æons of time since the individual "Spark of God" which is *you*, broke forth from the group-soul for freer expression of its Divinity.

Whenever you flashed a brilliant, clear colour—honest and unafraid, untinged by the mass-opinion—you have built an *atom* which is free to manifest as the physical perfection—which is *you*.

Whenever the pilgrim cravenly echoing mass-thought,

reacted as someone else deemed best, without that honest inward light of conviction (which alone should be the guide), a causation has started which will, in time, show one of those "misty spots" in the nebulous mass about you (which is your *aura* or the outpicturing of your soul's consciousness). In time this causation will manifest as a physical defect—a weakness—a disease.

Chrome-Therapy (Colour Healing) aims at re-establishing your colour-balance, or Divine birthright of Perfection, by breaking through these dams of error-thought, releasing the tension caused by "Colour-starvation," manifested in the physical *you*, and placing you once again where you may be "Captain of your Soul and Ruler of your Thought-children," as you bask in the beauty and comfort of Colour-treatments.

Within, there will be the stirring of your soul in response to the voice of your Higher Self—a self-revealed plan for a new way of thinking—a new life urge.

Do not neglect or delay in responding to this self-revealed *New Light*, for within its radiance you will find *perfect expression*, freedom, joy, and radiant living.

For the especial benefit of the peoples of Great Britain, at this time, I would mention the following treatment for shell- and bomb-shock:

It should be remembered that the violent percussions from shells and bombs produce colours of enmity, as seen in fierce struggle in battle, at times accompanied by sweeping uncontrollable emotions. These sudden emotions increase the vibrations of the Astral body so rapidly as to cause it to swing pendulum-like beyond the etheric double—its normal boundary of vibratory freedom or motion. In the case of people suffering from shell-shock these impacts have been violent enough to throw the astral completely out of equilibrium.

The radiant way to restore normalcy is first to place the patient in his or her colour of *Rest* using spiritual, mental or physical methods as the case may be. If a lamp is employed, start using the colour of *Rest* from five to eight minutes or a little longer, according to the reaction of the patient. Then give from three to five minutes under his or her colour of *Activity*, alternating these colours in this ratio for half an hour.

The next day slowly increase the *Activity* ray's duration until it equals the *Rest* ray. Throughout the days following increase the duration of both colours very gradually until, at the end of the first ten days' treatment, the entire treatment lasts a full hour.

When this goal has been reached each treatment should be closed by ten minutes spent in the colour of *Inspiration* until one day the re-alignment of the body will take place and the patient be restored.

I have found that the time required for this final accomplishment differs considerably and seems to depend largely upon the sensitivity of the patient, so that it really appears at times that the most serious cases are healed very quickly while the less serious sometimes take months.

Where there is not time or opportunity to learn the patient's exact colours before starting, it is safest to experiment by testing his or her reflexes while under Indigo, Lemon Yellow, or Violet, and assuming the colour stimulating the best response to be the colour of *Activity*. The testing of the reflexes of the patient will be readily understood by any nurse or, of course, physician.

Next test the patient's ability to relax under the rays of Green, Blue, or Violet, in the order named, and you will approximate the colour of *Rert*.

In this way you will learn to reseal the patient's etheric body, restore the shattered aura and re-establish the emotional and mental equilibrium.

Remember, whatever the disease being treated, it is through *Colour-breathing* that you draw into your atomic structure a certain permanence of Colour-balance, fixing the right colour and consciously making it impossible to respond to future circumstances with the wrong colour (thought). The lamp, or other means of Chrome-Therapy, will cure your distress or disease, but *permanent* perfection of expression *must* come from *your* conscious co-operation with the chrome-practitioner.

There are many methods of using Chrome-Therapy; some more or less successful in certain cases, but the treatments described in this volume have been proved to be most scientific, and have consequently produced the greatest number of permanent cures.

Each day I pray that Colour Awareness may free the body

centres of all of you in Europe, and illumine the Path of to-morrow's radiant attainment. Live, love, serve and *survive* through Colour—the Great Cosmic Tuning Fork, the *Master Control* of the New Race Vibration. With Colour's Blessings,

IVAH BERGH WHITTEN.

CALIFORNIA.
  October, 1940.

PREFACE

by THE AUTHOR

FOR many years I have felt that there was a great need for a comprehensive and practical text-book dealing extensively with the *application* of Colour. After all, of what avail is Colour Knowing without the technique of Colour Applying?

I have read many beautiful books, written (I gather from the quality of their expression), by equally beautiful souls; and other works have passed through my hands which have gathered theories, throwing out here and there a few practical but often unrelated hints. I do not doubt that they have all served their pioneer purpose of stimulating general interest in this radiant subject. As hors d'œuvres and apéritifs they have been excellent, but the whetted appetite of the novitiate student, I felt, would hardly feel quite satisfied. These works —with the exception of Dr. Edwin Babbitt's monumental work, "The Principles of Light and Colour"; and Dr. Iredell's splendid work, "Colour and Cancer"—have been all too slender reeds in this growing practical world that seeks a staff.

The fundamental laws and principles governing the cosmic energy we know as Colour have been ever present in Wisdom Teachings proclaimed by the Masters of All Ages, though beclouded in most men's minds until the days when the sun of our consciousness was strong enough to dispel the clouds of confusion.

To-day, research and invention, philosophy and psychology, biology and bio-chemistry, physics and metaphysics are all uncovering facets of the jewel of Colour Wisdom, so long buried in its shining completeness, to emerge as the new Science of Colour.

To present, enumerate, classify, tabulate and correlate even a tithe of such data in an essentially usable way so that the student might put his finger on chapter and verse at a moment's notice, has been the crying need. Enquiries from all over the world have shown this in their constant demand for a practical straightforward text-book outlining a definite technique.

Consequently my friend and teacher, Ivah Bergh Whitten,

who is putting forth the wonderful Master Lessons in Colour Awareness, consented to find time in a busy life of service, to write a book to be entitled "Using Colour", presenting a technique of the Masters. That work is still in the process of careful compilation and is on that account the more eagerly awaited and anticipated.

Owing to certain difficulties of publication and European distribution from America at this time, and in order to meet the pressing needs of students, and especially those of the world as it is to-day, I finally decided to collate the data of some years' research and experience, made possible through study, meditation, and the kindness of friends. I therefore present this MS., correlating most of the known with many new practical methods of colour-diagnosis and Colour Healing, to bridge the need until "Using Colour" may be in our hands and fruitfully employed by us all.

ROLAND HUNT.

Chapter I

INTRODUCTION

Colour Healing is a Divine Science.

It is not a cult, or fad, recently invented or discovered. It was used effectively in the Golden Age of Greece, and in the Healing Temples of Light and Colour at Heliopolis in ancient Egypt, and again, it was revered in the ancient civilizations of India and China. Throughout the ages there has always been the employment of the Colour Wisdom to establish poise and harmony; to soothe and sustain, to heal and restore, and to create anew. They were all expressions of the urge in the One Divine Creative principle in Light-waves.

Colour is, therefore, a Divine Force—nothing less!

To regard it, for one moment, as anything less would be like the woman who recalled only that electricity was something that heated her press iron. Whereas we know it is a cosmic energy that man has learned to harness to give artificial light, heat and cold, transport facilities and other services and comforts to the human family throughout the world.

Colour similarly offers its comforts and services to man, indeed, electrical and Light (Colour) waves have a common origin in the Sun power—the great comforter and energizer.

In America Professor Woods, Dr. C. S. Abbott, and Ellis L. Manning, physicist of the General Electric Company, independently of each other, have produced motors running entirely by Solar Power. In Colour Healing the White sunlight is used, in all its spectrum of Colour wavelengths, to run the motor organs of the human machine efficiently; not alone to restore the physical body, but to tone and refreshen the Mind and nourish the Spirit.

This wondrous Sun is one focal centre of God's Power in our zodiacal system—and in our human systems. The Energy-waves from the Sun create, sustain and renew Life in all kingdoms on our Earth and upon all other planets in the zodiac, which in turn reflect their vibratory rays on each other. The self-same principles that sustain Life in the cosmic system naturally sustain Man in his lesser, micro-cosmic system—in the working of the major glandular organs, or centres, of his body.

If through some failure in Cosmic Law and Order, the Earth were to be plunged into complete and continued darkness for but a few weeks, and then restored to Light, all vegetation would be found to have lost its colourful vitality, to have become anæmic, and would finally wither and disappear. There would correspondingly have been a similar effect on the health and vitality of Humanity. We all depend on Light more than is yet fully realized, for, as we see above, even our foods are densified chemical Light-waves, and this we shall refer to more fully presently.

Of all kingdoms of Life, the Human possesses the faculty of reasoning and the power to employ Will. Man has thus used his creative power to discover ways to use various groups of cosmic energy, such as electricity in lighting his physical darkness. He has thus extended his daily hours of usefulness.

On the other hand that same free-will has often ignored the value of light, and he has immured himself, and his brothers, in insufficiently lighted, cramped, houses in congested cities and towns.

Worse still he has, all too often, drawn the black-out curtains of ignorance and prejudice over his mental, emotional and spiritual understanding.

Through this negation of light we find many people suffering from a large variety of physical and nervous ailments—many of which originate in either mental or emotional perversion or inversion. Such people are plagued with all manner of inhibitions.

Broadly speaking there are two classifications for disease: (1) That which is infectious, or induced by wrong environment, *i.e.* through faulty working, living or climatic conditions, or in other words, having physical origin; (2) that which originates in the consciousness of the individual, *i.e.* in our emotional behaviour, mental attitudes, and spiritual outlook—or metaphysical in origin.

Colour has the beautiful and purposeful mission of alleviating both classes of dis-ease, not with the patchwork substitutes of drugs, but with the pristine power of Light, which works on *all* levels of our being. Truly, it is very largely due to our general inability to illumine our lives emotionally, mentally and spiritually, that we have loss of tone or disease physically.

We might put it that such people have misty spots in their consciousness which becloud their Inner Sun, the sunlight of their souls (Soul meaning Sol, or Sun). These blind spots, so to speak, screen off the inpouring of spiritual light, and where a habit, trait, vice or continued bias remains, the prolonged lack of nourishing light brings about a "light starvation" in certain parts of the physical body, and impairs the circulation of Life Forces through that part, resulting in a dis-eased organ, or possibly a malignant growth.

These negative spots in the health of the system are visible in the aura, or magnetic atmosphere of the patient, verily as dark spots, or blemishes—spots where the soul's light has failed to penetrate through to the physical to sustain it, resulting in a lowering of vitality, a decrease in vibration, a decay or disease.

Now our mental and emotional behaviourism is keyed to the seven major glandular centres in the human body, and continued mental or emotional stress, shutting off the soul's sustaining light, impairs one or more of those seven centres.

Again, these seven major centres in the body each have their own particular rate of vibration and absorb from the food we eat, the thoughts we think, the emotions we harbour, certain qualities or vibrations whose rate of frequency is identical respectively with each of the seven colours of the spectrum.

In other words, the White light (Christ-light) drawn into the consciousness of the soul is diffused into its seven component colours, each one being sent to sustain the centre to which it has an affinity. According to our stage in evolution we utilize our Ray-energy to build talents or vices; the one builds the consciousness of strength, the other dissipates it into the consciousness of disease. Only our wrongful or misguided habits, false reasoning, or violent emotions, prevent, or poison as the case may be, this circulation and deflect the diffused Ray-tinctured White light from its appointed dury.[1]

The primary and paramount necessity is therefore, obviously, to dissolve these self-made obstacles or dams, holding up our Divine supply, at whatever level they may have been constructed.

[1] See "What Colour Means to You," by Ivah B. Whitten, A.M.I.C.A.; also "Fragrant and Radiant Healing Symphony," by the Author.

Colour, objectively near at hand in our everyday lives is thus subjectively closer to our understanding—the one all-potent Cosmic Force that we may intelligently and readily apply to clarify these conditions and give release.

TABLE OF COLOUR-SOLARISED SUBSTANCES

(Based on Terminology in part suggested by Dr. Babbitt)

Prefix—signifying Colour	LUME signifies colour-solarized or artificial LIGHT	O signifies EAU colour-solarized WATER	GUM signifies colour-solarized GUM ARABIC	LAC signifies colour-solarized SUGARofMILK	SAC signifies colour-solarized SUGAR	SAL signifies colour-solarized SALT	GAS signifies colour-solarized AIR
Rubi (RED)	Rubilume	Rubigo	Rubigum	Rubilac	Rubisac	Rubisal	Rubigas
Orange (ORANGE)	Orangelume	Orangero	Orangum	Orangelac	Orangesac	Orangesal	Orangegas
Amber (YELLOW)	Amberlume	Ambero	Ambergum	Amberlac	Ambersac	Ambersal	Ambergas
Verd (GREEN)	Verdilume	Verdigo	Verdigum	Verdilac	Verdisac	Verdisal	Verdigas
Cerule (BLUE)	Cerulume	Ceruleo	Cerulegum	Cerulelac	Cerulesac	Cerulesal	Cerulegas
Indigo (INDIGO)	Indigolume	Indigolo	Indigum	Indigolac	Indigosac	Indigosal	Indigogas
Viole (VIOLET)	Violume	Violeo	Violegum	Violac	Violesac	Violesal	Violegas
Purpur (PURPLE)	Purpurlume	Purpuro	Purpurgum	Purpurlac	Purpursac	Purpursal	Purpurgas

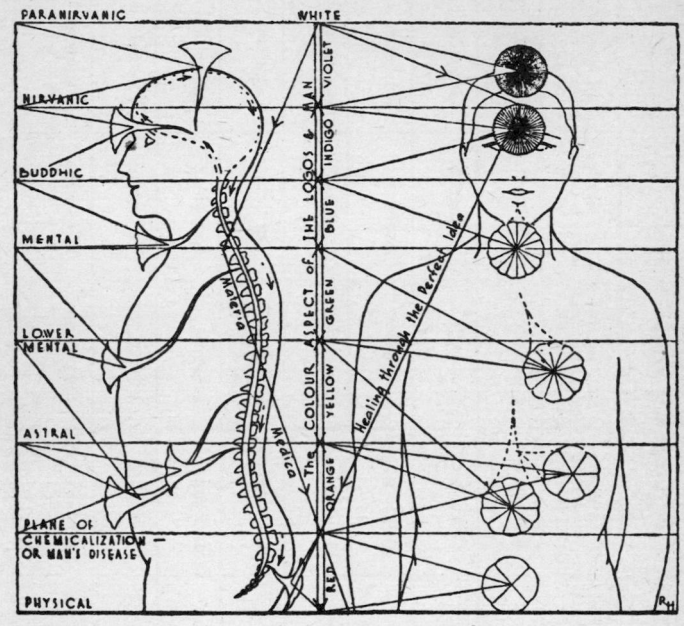

CHART showing:

(a) The Chakras—The Seven Doorways to Colour Healing.

(b) Healing through Colour, as compared with other methods of healing (from "What Colour Means to You," by Ivah B. Whitten, A.M.I.C.A.).

Chapter II

METHODS OF DIAGNOSIS

THERE are, in main, two methods of diagnosis. One is largely metaphysical—observing cause; the other is mostly physical —observing symptoms. Of these the first is paramount and absolute, for it sees to the root of the matter; the second is valuable to those without developed colour awareness, or etheric vision, serving chiefly to *classify* the complaint.

As the methods under number one are of primary importance, let us consider those first.

Metaphysical Methods of Diagnosis

The student seeking this information will doubtless understand that man is not merely a physical being—he has finer vehicles of expression through which his soul-force works, the physical body being the densest of them all.

The body most closely identified with the physical body is the etheric or sensational body; then of finer etheric substance is the Astral, emotional or desire body; interpenetrating this, is the Lower mental body or concrete mind; and transcending this again, is the Higher mental body; and in ascendancy over the mental bodies are the Spiritual, Intuitional, and Causal bodies.

It is thus evident that we have seven bodies within the one, the radiation from them all composing the aura,[1] or magnetic atmosphere. Herein is depicted in waves of light and colour, the physical, emotional, lower and higher mental and spiritual addendum of consciousness—the inhering talents, the deficiencies, the vibrant health or the weakness of disease.

To the advanced seer it is relatively easy to diagnose at which level, or in which body, originates the disease germ, and thus to treat at that level or in that body. Advanced seers, such as Ivah B. Whitten, A.M.I.C.A., can make such a diagnosis at a distance of many thousands of miles providing there is a vibrational link with the individual, such as a pressed flower that has been held in the hands.

[1] "What Colour Means to You, including What Your Aura Means to You," by Ivah B. Whitten, A.M.I.C.A.

23

However, not all clairvoyants are permitted to see the entire aura of a soul's consciousness. Only initiates, who are advanced, and highly trained seers working in perfect selflessness and purity of motive, are privileged upon occasion to see the soul bared to the causal body.

Nevertheless, very useful information may be derived by those able to observe health conditions at the emotional and mental levels, for these are the great breeding grounds of the germ-thoughts of our bodily complaints.

The data obtained by the seer, gifted with deep understanding of what is seen, have recorded information of first-hand accuracy and more valuable than any deductions arrived at by psychiatry or physiology alone.

For those who have not yet developed seership, there remain the following methods of diagnosis by observing the conditions further down the scale, on etheric and astral levels, by means of a Kilner Screen.

This screen is composed of two pieces of glass between which has been poured a solution of diocene, a liquid of indigo-violet colour, which, when looked through eliminates from vision all the coarser colours of the spectrum and sharpens the acuity of the observer.

This is advantageously used with a specially built diagnosing cabinet. In this the patient should be seated clad in but one garment, a thin straight-cut black silk robe. The cabinet should be shaped according to Diagram X, and the dimensions should be five feet wide at the front edge, four

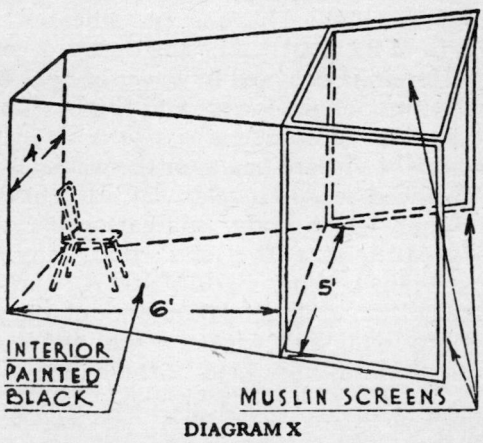

INTERIOR PAINTED BLACK

MUSLIN SCREENS

DIAGRAM X

feet at the back and six feet in depth. A stool should be provided upon which the patient sits erect and as far back in the cabinet as possible. Across the open front of this cabinet are attached and extended three-foot screens covered with unbleached muslin, and a drop screen of the same material. The side-screens are extended at an angle of about 115° on either side, whilst the drop screen bridges the two wings, thus forming a complete shield serving to soften intruding outside light and promoting better diagnostic vision. Then by the use of the diocene screen, the physical and emotional auras may be seen. It will probably take some practice to be able to detect the difference between the colour of Rest and the colour of Activity. The colour of Rest will be noticed to have a smooth flowing serene quality, while careful scrutiny will reveal the colour of Activity to possess a vital sparkling quality. According to the location of vibrancy or limpness of radiation in this "health-aura", as it is sometimes called, may be determined the health and efficiency of the various organs related to those parts.

The colour of Inspiration may not be seen through this screen, nor, as has already been mentioned, may the radiation of the higher bodies.

If the preparation of a diagnosing cabinet is not possible, then the healer wishing to diagnose through the Kilner Screen, should place the subject in a darkened room and after a few minutes gazing through the screen the healer will begin to observe the radiation from the etheric body.

Should the observance of the "health aura" only be practised, it would be well to check the result by psychological and astrological tests. The former may be gained by testing the subject's reactions—his preferences or dislikes—to different colours, e.g. in his clothing, in his living quarters or office, etc. Additional information may be gleaned by enquiry, whether he likes to see large masses of his preferred colours, and if he also likes to see them in the possession of others. Secondly, the casting of the subject's horoscope, ascertaining, which planetary influences are in the ascendency over him, often affords a good check to the "health-aura" diagnosis, although, it must be said, these data should not be considered absolute. In this connection it is well to remember that birth-date does not always fix the ego's Ray although it usually indicates it.

Physical Methods of Diagnosis

Lastly, there remain the methods of diagnosis, or checking, by observing the physical symptoms. These are particularly valuable in cases of emergency when immediate relief is very urgent.

It should be remembered that, on broad principle, there are but two principal colours, the heating Red and the cooling Blue-Violet, Green representing the middle point in between, the balance, or fulcrum. These are the outstanding colours of the rainbow.

Our aim, in broad diagnosis, is to discover which of the opposite colours is wanting in a certain body, and how to make up that balancing colour and thus remove the complaint.

To this end, we should observe the patient's habits, moods and reactions. For instance, if a man needs red in the system he would be inclined to be lazy, idle, sleepy, anæmic. He would lack appetite and be constipated, and so on. If a man requires the bluish end of the spectrum he would be hot-tempered, active, and be inclined to feverishness.

The Indian colour-healer, Jwala Prasada,[1] Munsiff of Benares, employs only the following physical methods of diagnosis. He says: "I have found from experience that the colour of four things decide what colour is wanting in a system: (1) The colour of the eye-balls; (2) The colour of

---

[1] Jwala Prasada says of himself: "In 1880 I was in search of something by which I could be of use to humanity at large. I had already become a tolerably fair magnetiser. This practice developed in me a general love for humanity and for the treatment of diseases. But I found that I could not attend to all my patients, who kept on increasing. Then I took to homeopathy. But after all, I found that both these systems of treatment are not such as to prevail in the long run, and I was in search of some such treatment that would offer real and lasting benefit to humanity. At last I came to have Babbitt's Health Manual (now out of print), in which I found the principles of Chromopathy recorded, and I have been practising this science ever since. I am now in a position to state that this treatment is to supersede all other treatments. It is at once the cheapest, the mildest and the most effective of all treatments known. It is especially suited to all who are spiritually inclined and I hope every lover of mankind will try to spread its principles among the general public."

the nails; (3) The colour of the urine; (4) The colour of the excrement.

"For instance, supposing a man wants Red colour, his eyes would be bluish, his nails would be bluish, his urine would be white or bluish, and his excrement would be white or bluish. If a man wants Blue colour, his eyes would be reddish, his nails abnormally reddish, his urine would be yellowish with, a tinge of red, or completely red, and his excrement would be yellow or red.

"Of course, it must be remembered that some people want a little red, some more red, while others want a little blue, and some more blue, and the frequency of the doses must be regulated by the degree of want of colour in the system. If a man shows of a sudden a large quantity of red colour in him and consequently a want of a proportionately large quantity of blue colour, as in cases of Cholera and Hydrophobia, the blue colour must be administered by repeated doses at short intervals.

"Sometimes it appears that a certain colour has accumulated in a certain place in the system, as in the case of boils, sore eyes, headaches, paralysis, etc., but in fact the whole system has that colour and it is only by its sudden outbursts at certain points that we are apprised of its accumulation. In such cases, it is always good to use both methods of treatment, internal (colour-solarized water) and external (coloured light).

"There are some points which sometimes deceive one in diagnosing the disease, and it generally happens with the colour of the eyes. The eyes may appear reddish and still the system may want red colour. This is due to weak persons working too much with their brains. The brain shows more heat than the other parts of the body, and it is due to over-exertion. But when the colours of the other three things are known the deception vanishes and we are able to know the wanting colour.

"In the case of children, the blue colour predominates in the eyes, as also in persons living in cold climates; but even in these cases the colours of the other three things settle the question. I may mention one particular thing which I have observed about the nails of the fingers. They show sometimes vertical lines in them, sometimes very thin and sometimes very thick. These lines indicate phlegm in the system *i.e.* want of red colour, and a little experience about these lines gives us a knowledge of the period of the disease. In almost all cases I have been able to fix the period of ailments with an unerring precision."

Chapter III
METHODS OF TREATMENT

WHERE there is disease, or deficiency in receiving the correct amount of Sunshine (or colour values), by one or more of the glandular centres, the lack may be supplied by inhaling, introducing or projecting, the required colour tones (*a*) directly into the physical body by means of correct food and solarized liquids, (*b*) into the physical counter-part, the etheric double, which immediately reflects physical health, or (*c*) into the soul's complete aura reaching *cause*, and arriving at change of consciousness and thus indirectly influencing physical health.

Colour-Solarized Treatment

In Chapter I we suggested the broad classification of diseases into two groups: (1) Physical in origin, and (2) Metaphysical in origin.

Let us suppose that diseases of the first group, then, have their origin in the physical system and then review the various "physical" methods available for treating by Colour. We will take the solarizing methods first.

During sunny summer days an ideal piece of equipment, if you have a fairly spacious garden, is a revolving sun-chalet.[1] This should be constructed much on the lines of the much-read-about revolving outdoor study used by Mr. Bernard Shaw. It enables the occupant to turn the hut so that it follows the course of the sun. The main difference in the Colour-Chalet is that the roof and one entire side should be made of removable vita-glass, over which any desired colour-screen may be drawn. In this way it is possible to catch the sun's rays, supercharged with Colour, at any angle of declivity or at any time of day.

Similarly, changeable colour-screens may be also fitted to the windows of a treatment room in the house, or in different rooms which catch the morning and afternoon sun.

A simple localizing device for utilizing the sun's rays is the tripod with Colour-Cone-Screens, or just colour-screens. These are fixed on an adjustable trombone arm sliding through a universal joint enabling the colour sunrays to be

[1] If space does not permit, then a miniature revolving colour-cabinet is a useful compromise.

focused on any body part. The patient reclines comfortably in an adjustable chair or portable couch, and canvas screens of a suitable height may, if needed, be employed to shut off chilling winds and ensure a measure of privacy.

Solar-Chrome Saline Rubs

In certain types of disease, such as Paralysis, in which physical or magnetic massage is generally advantageous, colour-charged salt-bags are beneficially used as valuable massaging accessories.

These salt-bags are made of double cheese-cloth and filled with two cupfuls of raw bran and half-a-cupful of Iodized or common salt. The bags are colour-charged by being placed in the sun, or lamp, radiation for one hour, before using. A full Rainbow range of colour salt-bags may be prepared by obtaining cloth of different colours or by cutting up the cheese-cloth, in the first instance, into seven lots, and dyeing each piece one of the spectrum colours.

Colour-Solarizing Fragrance-Fans

These are appealing accessories for those in invalid rooms, or for ladies residing in hot climates.

They are made out of organdie stretched and doubled over a light frame which finishes in a practical handle. In between the thicknesses of organdie, pot-pourri of flower petals is loosely filled. Organdie of various colours and pot-pourri of different Ray-flowers are used correlatively.[1]

When on the terrace or near a sunny window, the patient holds the colour-fan screen between her face and the Sun and wafts the cooling fragrant air towards her, enjoying a combined colour-fragrance tonic. Thus for example the violet organdie fan filled with pot-pourri of sweet violets offers a delightful way of taking Violegas.[2]

Diffused Sunshine in Diet

One of the most efficacious ways of restoring our colour-balance is through diet—through the foods we eat and the liquids we drink. All vegetables draw in the chemical and

[1] Further detailed in "Lighting Therapy and Colour Harmony", by the Author.
[2] See Table of Colour-Solarized Substances, facing page 20, also Violet Section.

light rays from the Sun, in different degrees according to their different natures and qualities.

Just as all individuals may be classified into seven main groups according to the Ray upon which they incarnate, so also may all vegetable-life be classified.

As it is a fact that we use up our own Ray-energy more quickly than any other, it is wise to include in our diet a slight favourable balance of our Ray vegetables. Thus those subjects of the Red Ray, predisposed to anæmia and other troubles of the bloodstream and circulation, should include iron-bearing vegetables such as beetroots, radishes, water-cress, red-cabbage and spinach, etc., and all the red-ripe fruits preponderantly in their menus, whilst those incarnating on the Violet Ray should favour those vegetables high in phosphoric content.[1]

It is not meant that we should become faddy in our food, but that we should keep a discriminative eye on the classes of food preponderating in causing deficiencies or excess, or balance in our particular make-up. The phrase is now trite but its truth evermore revealed, that "we are what we eat ——," and to the quotation we might well add, "——and drink." All fruits from which drinks are prepared can be similarly classified and employed to the benefit of our health.

It is all too obvious that fruits and vegetables are the highest forms of material food on our planet; they draw the greater part of their electrical energy direct from the sun's rays, and even the chemicals of the soil from which the roots draw secondary magnetic energy, are sustained by the same solar and planetary power. As the leaves and fruits are matured and ripened by direct contact with the solar rays they form finer foods than those from beneath the ground. "Indeed, the organic and mental characteristics which each individual inherits may be changed by the mode of life, the refinement of chemical substances in foods, the climate and the physiological and moral disciplines," says Dr. Alexis Carrel.

As man ascends in the scale of evolution, developing a finer body through a finer consciousness he will arrive at such results largely through finer foods. From the dense physical consciousness supported by equally dense foods crea-

"Colour in Diet," by the Author (in preparation).

ting much ash and involving cellular decay in his system and advancing old age through his inability to throw off the great accumulation of waste, man, we are told, will evolve to an awakened awareness of the nature and relationship of his physical make-up to that of Nature. As he grows towards the choice of foods carrying the maximum cosmic and solar energy with the least amount of ash, he will extend and dynamize his consciousness and the active span of his life.

Some yogis have brought this discrimination to a fine art by drawing in all their needs *direct* from the Divine Cosmic Solar-Energy, dispensing with any of the *densified* forms of solar-light-waves in the bulk of foods. With the knowledge of such cosmic laws of life they are able to control the elements within and outside of themselves, performing seemingly miraculous feats and tests of endurance, and living for hundreds of years.

In the West we have amongst others the case of Professor Ehret, who suffered from indigestion and anæmia since boy-hood, eventually finding relief and sustenance in vegetables and fruit juices, and finally he said good-bye to even inter-mittent indigestion by giving up dense foods altogether. He went on observed fasts for fifty days at a time, and then would outstrip young meat-eaters at mountain climbing. By resting the physical assimilative apparatus, he had opened the cosmic medullary mouthpiece in his higher bodies.

This is exactly the way in which the Angelic Evolution is sustained—through the nourishment of Cosmic Light and Colour, which is not only their nourishment but their very language.[1] This is not a fundamental principle unique to one kingdom of Life, it is a cosmic principle pertaining to *all* Life, and when we humans realize of what our finer bodies and true foods consist, we shall largely free ourselves from the very possibility of disease.

A Celestial Materia Medica

It has been said that evolution progresses at the pace of the slowest, and it is such that need the greatest helping hand, for the good of all. Let us therefore return to the subject of liquid diet. This may be surcharged with the beneficent colour-solar energy before consuming if we will but stand the

---

[1] "The Coming of the Angels," by Geoffrey Hodson, F.T.S.

juices out in the sunshine for a few minutes in a colour jar. The colour of the jar selected should be the same as the Ray of the fruit, to bring them back to freshness and their correct tone.

Various other foods and substances are very suitable carriers of Colour-Solar-Energy, *viz.* Sugar, Sugar of Milk, Gum Arabic, etc., and may be surcharged in the manner above.

Rainbow Healing

In the case of colour-solarized water (Colour Water, or "sun-kissed water" as a student has charmingly called it) this is one of the finest, easiest, and cheapest ways of taking Colour into the system. It is literally and truly the essence of Rainbow Healing. Just as after the Deluge, the rainbow was God's bright promise to the world, so colour scintillating potently through pure water offers Rainbow Healing full of promise and satisfaction for a sickly world. The basic principles were introduced into materia medica, in comparatively modern times, by Dr. Edwin Babbitt, M.D., LL.D., who achieved great results. The very natural efficacy of Hydrochromatic treatment has had great appeal and result in such countries as India and California.

Dr. Babbitt forecast many years ago, that a Celestial Materia Medica would eventually be built up from Colour-charged substances. He says: "We have seen that every style of potency and substance is found in the most refined form in the different colours of sunlight. In the course of thousands of experiments with chromo-jars and lenses, it has been demonstrated that a new and remarkable healing power has been brought before the world. Water is the most practical substance for use in these jars, or hollow lenses, and it is medicated according to the colour, by letting the sun shine into it. Sugar of Milk, sugar and pulverized gum arabic, being nearly neutral, constitute good vehicles for taking luminous charges of *any* colour desired."

To refer easily to substances thus colour-solarized, the author, upon the inspiration of Dr. Babbitt, has prepared a table of suitable terminology. This nomenclature can be learned in a few minutes, and as we now have the exact significance of every colour, it forms the basis of a true science.

Another very important application of this system of refined therapeutics, is the inhalation of colour-charged *air*, which is signified by the affix *gas* (see Table, column 8). The only *normal* medicine for the lungs is air, and as the lungs are the fountain-head of blood purification and vitalization, such inhalation must be immensely important.[1]

Knowing that Blue light is one of the great antiseptics of the World, free from all poisonous influences which are so common with other antiseptics, it is expected that Cerulegas will bring about a new era in the treatment of pulmonary consumption and other tubercular diseases.

Artificial Sunlight

Next in the scale of values comes the colour-therapy lamp so useful for treatment in the clinic, in the home and at night-time.

The most elaborate of electrical colour-therapy apparatus, though simple in use, is the colour-treatment-cabinet, or Electro-Thermolume. This is constructed somewhat along the lines of a Turkish bath, except that treatment comes from a light-source at the front of the cabinet over which colour screens may be fixed and changed, so that a veritable colour-bath may be obtained.

The most generally used type of equipment is the colour-therapy standard lamp, which enables the patient to receive specific colour treatment sequence upon any particular body part. Treatment is best received in a darkened room with the subject entirely relaxed upon a couch covered with a sheet only. The lamp, or lamps, are then arranged in position beneath the sheet covering the patient, so that the direct rays may be absorbed without hindrance. For those who travel about considerably, those of no settled abode, a folding-type of lamp has been devised which packs flat into the suitcase, and so takes up very little room.[2]

Those who may be contemplating permanent residence in a new home, planning lighting and plumbing fixtures, might well consider constructing a hydro-chrome shower. This may be made by fixing seven coloured bulbs (ranging the spectrum) encased in glass above the water shower in the roof of

[1] See the use of Cerulegas, in the Blue Ray Section, page 83.
[2] "Lighting-Therapy and Colour-Harmony," by the Author.

a glass-enclosed shower cabinet. The bulbs should be fixed in the pattern of spokes from the hub of a wheel. The desired colour is switched on and the rays percolate through the descending water shower. What brighter tonic to start the day, or to freshen up in the evening, than a Rainbow Shower.

In some Hydros they have what is called a "Medical Shower". This is composed of a central shower above the head, and pipes led down the four corners of the glass-sided cubicle, releasing side, front, and back showers all the way down on to the entire body, and up from the very floor to the root of the spine. The secondary showers are so positioned that they play upon and stimulate all the functionary organs and centres of the body. If behind each of these showers a light-source were fixed of the correct colour for each of the organic centres, what a tonic Rainbow shower would be provided.

[In relation to diagnosing and treatment we would draw the reader's attention to the Drown Diagnostic and Treatment instrument, the invention of Dr. Ruth Drown, which diagnoses and treats Fourth Dimensionally, i.e. attunement is made through a sample of blood sent to the operator from which health diagnosis of the entire body is made, and treatment transmitted regardless of distance or time intervening. This remarkable New Age instrument is referred to in more detail in "The Fifth Dimension", by Vera Stanley Alder, published by Rider.]

Universal Breathing Affirmation

O Thou Radiant Spirit of Divine Love,
Enter my Inner consciousness;
O Thou Spirit of Divine Love,
Dwell in my Heart;
That Love may make Radiant—
Each Thought,
Each Word,
Each Deed,
Ever shining,
As my Brothers' Beacon,
Radiating
Joy—
Peace—
Power!

From "What Colour Means to You,"
by Ivah B. Whitten.

In the Alps there is oft-times a Dawn or Sunset glow on the snowy expanse of Peaks. Visualize this warming Pink glow as spreading over the entire Earth and all its inhabitants. Inhale as from the glowing Heights; exhale the radiance and goodwill far over the Horizon. The last part should not be forgotten, as without goodwill towards all, you render Healing ineffective and impermanent.

Chapter IV

TREATING CONSCIOUSNESS

Colour Breathing

IT is recommended that in all the above methods of treatment, and in those shortly to be described, the patient should co-operate in receiving treatment, wherever possible. This is very important if permanent results are to be obtained. Such receptivity may be promoted if the patient before and during treatment, and at other times such as upon rising in the morning and on retiring at night, practise Colour Breathing, *i.e.* realizing that Colour is pouring out upon him from the sunshine, the very earth, or from the treatment lamp in beneficent radiation, awaiting only his active awareness to become increasingly and permanently beneficial.

Therefore, he should practise the inhalation, and visualization, of these rays, breathing them into the body and mind as needfully and purposefully as the very air we unconsciously yet needfully draw into the lungs.

A simple mantra or affirmation attuned to the colour being used is found greatly helpful in this connection.

This Colour Breathing is found to be most exhilarating and uplifting because it affects and expands the consciousness to unmindfulness of irksome earthly troubles and sorrows. The refreshment is as effective as deep breathing is after habitual shallow breathing, only more so. The subject feels the glow of life and peace in mind and subsequently in body.

Universalizing the Breath

It is most natural and simple thing in the world to breathe in the things we want from the life of the macrocosmic system into the microcosmic life of our bodily system. The larger macrocosmic atmosphere is but an extension and expansion of our own microcosmic atmosphere—the Life-Force of our Father-Mother-God.

To realize the depth and fulness of the Divine Life in our being we should deliberately expel the dead, outworn things which we have harboured through our shallow breathing, shallow thinking and living, and breathe in deeply all the vital, pulsating ethers awaiting to float beneficently into our being, through the connection of our breath-life with The

Divine All-Health ether which encircles us—for ether is the atmosphere of the Spirit.

Here is a simple way to start breathing vitally. Sit well back in a straight-back chair with the spine erect, before your window, lightly but comfortably clad, preferably facing East. Then expel all air from the lungs and stomach as you bend forward, relaxing the body into limpness, arms dangling. Then breathe in slowly, straightening up the spine, concentrating the attention in between the eyebrows. At full inhalation hold the breath counting from 1 to 12 according to your own speed and comfort, realizing the breath is refreshing and recharging every cell in the body with new life, imparting to the mind freedom from all limitation, as you thus nourish your physical, your mental, and all your finer spiritual vehicles. Repeat the exercise twice.[1]

By thus breathing we can visualize outselves, truly, into sevenfold living. These complete breaths raise our bodily vibrations until we are able subjectively to unite with everything in the universe around us.

Then, to discard from the consciousness every vestige of the old conditions, to dissolve all thoughts of limitation (the cause of disease in the physical body) begin serenely and rhythmically to breathe deeply to a Universal affirmation, visualizing the radiant Peachy tint of Universal Love, and then extend your mental horizon until it embraces the Universe.

The mantra by Ivah Bergh Whitten, A.M.I.C.A., on page 37 has been found widely useful this way.

Then prepare for the specific treatment to follow, by breathing to the Colour Affirmation keyed to your prescription needs. (See the initial page to each of the sections on the Seven Colour Rays.)

When being treated with any one of the first three magnetic colour Rays, i.e. Red, Orange, and Yellow, visualize drawing in the warming cosmic breath up from the Earth through the very soles of your feet upwards to the solar plexus. When breathing in the last three electrical Rays, i.e. the Blue, Indigo, and Violet, breathe in the cooling colour from the heavens downwards; and Green, at the fulcrum,

[1] See "Scientific Healing Affirmations," by Paramhansa Yogananda, A.B.

between heaven and earth, breathe in horizontally as from fresh green countryside in the sunshine after the rain.

In the following sections of this book general colour treatment is outlined for the use of all the Rays. But it should be remembered that treatment becomes individual and unique when once we know our own Ray vibration, within which we find (1) our colour of Inspiration; (2) our colour of Activity, and (3) our colour of Rest. When in possession of this vital information we should learn to breathe deeply of our colour of Inspiration in the early morning, when developing ideas, planning, writing, or conceiving or working in the fields of Art. We should breathe in our colour of activity before and when doing the practical, energetic tasks of our daily lives, and we should breathe in our Colour of Rest when day is done.[1]

This gives the individualized uniqueness to Colour Healing. It will be realized presently, that one complaint can take on different shapes in different individuals. It is through these individual soul-colours that subtle, accurate treatment may be formulated.

The tremendous amount of wonderful work that can be done with Colour on mental levels is as yet barely understood. When we realize that every thought we think out-pictures in the aura as a blended flash of brilliant colour, we appreciate that colour is the very medium of our every thought expression. The symbology of colour teaches us the characteristic quality, or virtue, inherent in each tone of Colour, and if we would possess that quality or virtue in our consciousness we should take pains to introduce that particular tint into our lives, i.e. into our environment through our home furnishings, our dress, our home lighting—for this is the atmosphere we mentally breathe in and build into our own make-up.

A knowledge of the Colour Wisdom helps to dissolve the prejudicial bias of the mind, breeds a wider tolerance of the peculiarities of those incarnating on Colour Rays different from our own, and thus prevents that literal hardening of the heart and crystallization of mind and body that culminates in old age.

A dear lady, known to the author as a user of Colour for many years, recently went to a doctor for a confirmatory

[1] "Colour Breathing," by Ivah B. Whitten.

physical examination. The M.D. exclaimed: "Well, you must have something in that Colour of yours! I know you are over sixty, and I also know some of the hardships you have been through since the depression, but you have the body of a woman half your age, a remarkable body in the circumstances, very!" As the mind keeps a flexible texture so does the physical body likewise; one is the projection of the other.

Our environment creates the consciousness which induces the quality of our health, just as much as we build our environment from the very thoughts we think. It works both ways.

It is from this standpoint that Colour Psychology is being employed in our hospitals, universities, schools, sanatoriums, asylums, and in factories and workshops, so that we may live and work with greater ease, and freedom from the various impediments and accidents in life.

Dr. Donald Laird, Professor of Psychology at Colgate University, in a recent report confirms that certain colours in bedrooms cause insomnia, and that bright clothes and surroundings have a remarkable effect upon backward children. This is but one professional instance of the many ways we may employ Colour to remove the inertia, the backwardness of mental and bodily disease—they are legion!

"Perhaps the frontiers of the organs of the body are not where we believed them to be," says Dr. Carrel. "Each state of consciousness, it would seem, has a corresponding organic expression, and determines true pathological changes. Emotions determine the dilation of contraction of the small arteries through the vasomotor nerves; they are therefore accompanied by changes in the circulation of the blood in tissues and organs. Pleasure promotes circulation, causing the skin of the face to flush. Anger and fear, often contractile emotions, turn it white. Thus envy, hate, fear, when these sentiments are habitual, are capable of starting organic changes and genuine diseases. Mental and moral unbalance are the remote causes of colitis and the accompanying infections. On the other hand, certain spiritual activities may also cause anatomical as well as functional modifications of the tissues and organs. These organic phenomena are observed in various circumstances, among them being the state of prayer or affirmation—an absorption of consciousness in the contemplation of a principle both permeating and transcending our world. Such a psychological state is not intellectual: it is incomprehensible to philosophers and scientists and inaccessible to them. But the serene and simple seem to feel God as easily as the heat of the Sun, or the kindliness of a friend. Such facts are of profound significance. They show the reality of certain relations of still unknown nature, between the psycho-spiritual and organic processes. They prove the objective importance of spiritual activities which hygienists, physicians, educators and sociologists have almost always neglected to study. They open up immense new regions to man of a hitherto unknown world."[1]

Spiritual Colour Healing

The wonder of Colour is that it is not effective just on lower physical planes, as is materia medica to some degree, nor effective merely on mental and emotional planes as is Psychiatry; nor effective alone on Spiritual levels as with Faith healing—it works on *every* plane. The reason for this complete effectiveness is in the fact that Colour is a Divine Power that works through and in us, in every gland, in every cell of brain and body—and in every environment outside the body. Yet its greatest effectiveness is upon the spirit of man, in its influence upon the consciousness, the habitual thoughts, in which lie the seeds of our health and well-being.

When it is fully realized that disease in man, and the world, for the most part originates in consciousness and *only later* manifests in physical form; that our thought-waves radiate out as Colour, and that Colour applied to our environment and mental-atmosphere can change our mental outlook on Life—it must be admitted that Colour applied to the highest or causal levels, is of absolutely paramount importance.

Thus, in the spiritual use of Colour lies the greatest virtue —and the widest field of glorious service. Essentially, there is no basic need for any physical equipment, for spiritual healing transcends the material. Nevertheless, with many colour-healers spiritual healing augments physical and mental treatments, one often involving the other. The only basic requirements for spiritual colour-healing are those of

[1] "Man the Unknown," by Dr. Alexis Carrel.

soul-qualities in which the key quality is Selflessness, that invaluable asset to the work—and, a cone-pointed mind, capable of concentration.

Those drawn to this sphere of Colour Healing usually have developed Awareness,[1] possessing the ability to see in the higher odic, or spiritual octave of light-waves, corresponding to some extent with the lower octave absorbed by the physical eyes.[2] They have their inner eye opened and can draw the waves of Cosmic Colour Power to them, and by a concentrated effort of one-pointed Will[3] send out and direct the healing radiancy to any subject near or far. It matters not if the patient be thousands of miles distant physically, for, since cosmic Colour travels in the fourth dimension[4] it is received practically instantaneously if the patient is aware and receptive. If the distant patient is busily otherwise engaged, a compelling colour signal may be flashed into his consciousness to suggest a few quiet minutes of receptivity; or, alternatively the treatment may await him in the magnetic atmosphere of his home, till moments of repose are more opportune. When a suitable relaxation period occurs the treatment is then absorbed.

Naturally, the finer the sensitivity and capability of "attunement" of the recipient, the more comprehensive and permanent will be the result, but even in those of grosser natures treatment leaves a definite beneficial, if not lasting, effect.

When, eventually, with individual self-realization, aware-

[1] See "Lessons in Colour Awareness," by Ivah Bergh Whitten, A.M.I.C.A.

[2] See "Experiments in Magnetism," by Baron von Reichenbach; also "The Principles of Light and Colour," by Dr. Edwin Babbitt, M.D., LL.D.

[3] A beneficial exercise, when the student is able to see and control etheric Colour, is then to *will* the accumulated radiant colour to dissolve into a glassful of fresh water. The water thus becomes potently colour-charged for drinking or other healing purposes.

[4] "The Fourth Dimension," by Alexander Horn.

"The Fifth Dimension," by Vera Stanley Alder, and the research work of Dr. Ruth Drown, whose diagnostic and treatment instruments enable fourth dimensional treatment of the subject by Colour-irradiation from one's own source of supply of which one becomes fundamentally conscious. Thus the patient does not seek or depend upon some means of healing outside himself, but draws upon the cosmic forces within.

ness and sensitivity are balanced by understanding and control, we should reach the stage where we can weed our own garden, and plant only the spiritual blossoms of soul fragrance. Then we shall have reached the turning point, the spiritual rebirth, the reclamation of the kingdoms of the spirit within us, and make good the ancient injunction: "Man, heal thyself!"

Healing Colour-Breathing Affirmation
RED RAY

O Ruby Rays,
Flow through me,
Flow through me,
And Energize,
My bloodstream;
My bloodstream.

. . .

O Ruby Rays,
Stimulate,
Activity, Activity;
And instil
Iron Stamina,
Staunch Stamina.

. . .

O Ruby Rays,
Recharge my Will,
With Thy Goodwill,
For Health and Joy,
For Me and All——
I will *Fulfil.*

Breathe in these warming, vitalizing, magnetic Ruby Rays, as from the very molten heart of the Earth, up through the feet and legs to the affected spot.

Imagine the core of the earth as a glowing Ruby, or just visualize the lively Ruby Jewel at your feet, flashing out its radiant power and comfort, upwards to and through you.

Chapter V

RED

METALS radiating Red rays: Iron, Rubidium, Titanium, Bismuth, Zinc, Copper (the latter also radiates its complementary colour, Green).[1]

Chemicals, Elements and Gases: Potassium, Ferric Oxide, Ferrous Tri-oxide, Ammonium Carbonate, Bromine, Slaked Lime,[1] Hydrogen, and various alkalines.

The best glass to use for treatment purposes contains some of the above mineral substances.

Foods: Beetroot (tops and roots), Radishes, Red Cabbage, Watercress, Spinach, Aubergine; most deep red skinned fruits; black cherries, red currants, red plums, etc. etc.

Typical Diseases to which Red Ray subjects are prone: Ailments of the bloodstream, Anæmia, Physical Debility and Lassitude, Colds, Circulatory Deficiencies, Paralysis, Moronic cases, etc.

Characteristics of Red: Red has been called the "Great Energizer", the "Father of Vitality", because of its immense elementary effect upon the physical constitution of man. As an animating force for the blood Rubigas and Purpurgas are excellent. Red is heating; it warms the arterial blood, thus promoting circulation. The culmination of the heat rays (thermal or Infra-Red) lies considerably beyond the Red, according to Professor Robert Hunt. Red is very rich in calorific rays; it is alkaline, non-electric, non-stringent.

Locality and Affinity: Red controls the Root Chakram, or Coccygeal Centre, at the base of the spine (and also the lower limbs), which governs the vitality of the physical body, particularly the creative, procreative and restorative processes.

Treatment with Red stimulates this centre, causing adrenalin, stored in the ductless glands under its control, to be released into the bloodstream. Under the Red Light (Rubilume) the hæmoglobin corpuscles multiply in the blood and with the increased energy liberated, the bodily temperature is raised, the circulation extended and in-

[1] Red radiates predominantly, or in some cases equally, from these metals and substances. Several secondary colours, however, are often present. This note applies in principle to all the materials classified elsewhere in this book.

vigorated, dispersing lassitude and mucous-forming diseases inherent in chronic colds and chills.

Red is therefore useful in removing dormant or sluggish conditions. It expands and activates what has been contracted and held by an undue influence of chilling, stringent blue.

It is well to appreciate how correct diet aids the average person to benefit from Colour treatment.

Let us consider for a moment the disease of Anæmia: Materia Medica advocates Iron. This may be taken in organic form, *i.e.* in vegetable and fruit foods rich in iron salts.

A finer way of absorbing Iron is direct from the mineral rays of the Sun upon the body, preferably supercharged through a Red screen, or by inhaling Rubigas.

It is additionally recommended that each day several tumblerfuls of Red Solarized Water (Rubigo)—the Red mineral rays of the Sun dissolved in water—be taken regularly between meals.

Now let us consider what takes place physiologically when, say, Coloured Light treatment is applied.

When a beam of Red Light (Rubilume) is projected on the body, the etheric and physical body assimilates a certain amount of the red rays, and the latter decompose the salt crystals in our system. The Red Rays form Ions. These ions are minute particles which are carriers of the electromagnetic energy in our bodies. When the beam of Rubilume hits the ferric salt crystal, *i.e.* a particle donsisting of iron and salt, then it splits up this crystal into its component parts, namely, iron and salt, the iron being assimilated by the blood while the salt is discharged from the body. So the system is strengthened.

The releasing, expanding, and energizing power of Red is invaluable in curing partial and total paralysis; local paralysis being curable by Rubilume thrown on the diseased part. In this connection it should be remembered that mentally, Red urges physical *action* to overcome inertia or contraction. It is wilful, assertive, and banishes the sense of limitation and incapacity to cope with things. It promotes cheerfulness and initiative.

Spiritually, Red strengthens Will-power and courage, overcoming faintheartedness and lack of one-pointed Faith.

All play their part in the soul's battle to achieve freedom from bodily limitations.

Anæmia: Cases of Anæmia are treated in the following manner:—As in all treatments, the healer first of all mentally surrounds the patient with the Peachy Universal tint, through affirmation.

If the patient shows willingness to co-operate, he is asked to use the Universal breathing affirmation, followed by the Red Ray breathing affirmation every morning and evening, adapting the latter, if need be, to his particular complaint, thus willing the beneficent rays to do their work—to rebuild, or release, new health and activity in the body.

With this underlying awareness the patient is placed on a predominantly Red diet, i.e. a diet of mainly Red Ray vegetables and fruits containing iron; and he is allowed to drink freely of Rubigo in between meals.

When taking Light treatment, the patient lies flat upon a prepared couch with a sheet covering him. Rubilume is then projected from about six inches distance, upon the soles of the feet, whilst a second lamp of Orangelume is focused on the spleen for thirty minutes.

On sunny days it is recommended that whenever possible, noonday treatments should be included, using the Sun-power through small red screens or discs upon the soles of the feet, and breathing in the ruby rays.

During treatment the projections from the lamp or sun-disc should be gradually raised from the soles of the feet to the ankles, then calves, following to the knees. Afterwards up to the thighs, at a glancing angle towards the root chak-ram, resting from five to ten minutes at each location.

Treatment is finished off with ten minutes under the Green (Verdilume) or Blue light (Cerulume) to counteract any undesirable, or irritating, psychological effects.

In America several cases of paralysis have been treated, in the incipient stages, where patients could not walk, feeling their feet and lower limbs to be too heavy.

Paralysis: usually originates in the mental or emotional bodies, the patient having suffered shock or frustration through some acute or prolonged experience. So firstly, there must be some new absorbing interest.

Metaphysically, paralysis begins with this mental or emotional confusion—a not knowing which step to take next.

Gradually the fear and perplexity become so aggravated that the subject fears to take *any* initiative in any direction whatsoever. So he takes none! The door to all active interests seems closed with the result that, confused and unable to cope with the situation, the motor-nerves refuse to give orders. To restore the fundamental initiative therefore, new and practical interests must be found, and opened up.

"I have found the best results in adjusting the mental attitude, when the patient is unaware of its relation to the cure," says Ivah Bergh Whitten, A.M.I.C.A. "Yellow, in the initial stages of treating the mentality, is often helpful towards inspiring the mind with fresh initiative, and the inhalation of Ambergas is recommended.

"When the lock against motion is released, it only remains for Colour, the Great Cosmic Tuning-Fork, used specifically, to attune the new inflow of nerve force."

Allow the patient to drink Purpuro freely between meals, then commence Light treatment as follows:

"Have the patient lie face-downwards upon the couch, and start at the base of the spine with the Magenta Light (Purpurlume). Focus it on the Root Chakram for fifteen minutes.

"Then slowly move up the spine to the fifth dorsal vertebra, which is directly back of the Solar Plexus—move to this vertebra so slowly that five minutes is consumed in so doing.

"Next treat the feet leaving the Purpurlume focused on the soles for fifteen minutes.

"Then, if both legs are affected, each great sciatic nerve should be treated with Purpurlume, allowing the light to play upon the back of the legs in an upward direction.

"Then change to Rubilume treating the knees, shins and feet together for ten minutes.

"Proceed by switching to Indigolume, focusing the light for five minutes upon the Solar Plexus. Then slowly move the Indigolume up to the Power Centre in the throat, focusing it there for a further five minutes before changing to Cerulume for ten minutes.

"After twelve treatments have been given the patient will be able to follow the Ray work by visualizing the Life Force flowing through every atom.

"At this stage, the egoic Ray Colour of the patient should

be known and employed in order to seal the new inflow of energy, that it may not be dissipated.[1]

"It will take about three months for a complete cure, maybe longer, but the red-magenta rays may be stopped after the first eight weeks, in very bad cases, or five weeks in less acute instances. As the Ruby Ray stimulates adrenalin, it will of course be seen that an overdose is not wise.

"Impress upon the patient that he *can* be well, that he *can* do things."

Paralytic cases of long-standing invariably arrive at a quicker cure when spiritual colour healing and etheric massage are added to the solarized water and Light treatment. "Magnetic massage with many downstrokes for motor-paralysis, and upstrokes for sensory paralysis, would be doubly good," says Babbitt. There is an instance on record where one such case arrived helplessly in a wheel-chair, and after but the third treatment he astonished his homefolks by getting up by his own effort, walking out of doors and vigorously mowing the lawn. A thing he had *wanted* to do.

Consumption: Dr. Pancoast records a remarkable case of the treatment by Colour of tuberculosis *in the third stage*, with both lungs involved, "the left hepatized with mucous râle through the upper third, and crepitation in the apex of the right lung; sputa copious; her expectoration was a yellowish, ropy and frothy mucous and pus; she had severe nightsweats, and chills, followed by fever and flushed cheeks." Dr. Pancoast explains that her parents and most of the family had died of consumption. He continues: "I placed Mrs. H. under red baths regulated by the effects produced. In two weeks, improvement began to manifest itself in her symptoms; in another week the mucous râle became sub-mucous, then successively a crepitant and a bronchial, soon respiration was resumed through the entire left lung, and the crepitation apex of the right lung disappeared; expectoration improved and the cough became less frequent and distressing; with the improvement in these symptoms the chills and fever and the dyspnœa disappeared and her strength rapidly increased; in two months and a half, the only remaining trouble was a slight cough arising from an irritated throat!" He concludes, "in an active and extensive practice covering

[1] In this way the subject's mental (Inspirational) colour may be used first, and then his physical colour of Activity.

more than thirty years, we have never known or heard of a case of consumption at so advanced a stage successfully treated. Her recovery was complete."

Dr. Babbitt quotes a letter from Mme. Camille Lemaitre, St. Florentin, France, regarding the effect of red-solarizing different foods: "I used red glass over a yellow vase so as to act upon bread, milk and fruits. For many years I have had a very sensitive taste. After they had remained some time under a bright sun, I felt a spicy and peppery taste on my tongue from them. That which had been sun-charged had acquired a particular quality. My digestion became very active. Thus, under the red and yellow rays, the bread which in its ordinary state seemed heavy, became expanded and very much lighter. The milk which was exposed under a bright sun for three hours was made much more digestible. What an advantage this will be for the stomachs of infants who are supported upon certain kinds of milk when not able to receive the natural supply."

Infantile Paralysis: This widely prevalent disease may be readily cured by hydro-chromopathic means. The Ruby shower should be employed, followed by Rubilume and Rubisal treatment, and it would be well if the Ruby breathing affirmation were introduced. Nurse Kenny of Melbourne, Australia, has had unusual success with colour-hydropathic methods, employing colour-psychology to the extent that even the attendant nurses are required to dress in the appropriate colour.

It should always be remembered, however, that the heating and excitable Red rays are detrimental to the majority of nervous complaints, as they prove too stimulating to the point of alarming irritation. With emotionally susceptible patients they should be used with extreme caution and smoked glasses are often advisable when treating generally with Red.

In its flame tints, Red is sometimes beneficial, psychologically, to those suffering from depression and deep melancholia, as its warming activity arouses them from the depths of contemplative despair, inspiring fresh courage, will-power and initiative.

However, in many of these mental-emotional cases, it is often wiser to substitute Orange for Red, and it is this vibrant freeing Colour whose healing power and virtues we will next consider.

ORANGE RAY

O Freeing Orange,
O Buoyant Rays—
Float in me,
Float in me—
Salving, Restoring,
Conscious Will,
Conscious Energy,
Above all limits
Of Bodily mind.

. . .

O Warming Orange
Dispel All Chills
And Kindred Ills—
In me Health thrills.

. . .

O Lifting Orange,
Transmuting Rays,
'Waken, unfold,
My Budding Powers;
Bring me Wisdom's
Bright new Powers,
Bright New Powers.

Just as the Sun enlightens and warms the Earth—so both Sun and Earth enlighten and warm the children of Earth. Breathe in its Wisdom-Light. Mentally send the Red part of the ray to all parts of your physical body, and in the same way send the Yellow part of the ray up to your Mind.

Think of the Red part of the ray as making you feel strong and energetic; and think of the Yellow part as making your mind dynamic, alert, and Good-natured. The last part should not be forgotten, as without Goodwill towards All you render healing ineffective, impermanent.

Chapter VI

ORANGE

METALS radiating Orange: Selenium, Iron, Calcium, Nickel, Zinc (not advised for healing uses), Rubidium, Manganese.

Chemicals, Elements, Gases: Carbon, Oxygen (slightly), and many Alkalines.

Best glass to use in treatment contains Selenium and Uranium Oxides, Manganese and Red Lead.

Foods: Most orange skinned vegetables and fruits; Carrots, Swedes (Rutabagas), Pumpkin; Oranges, Apricots, Persimmons, Mangoes, Cantaloupes, Tangerines, Peaches.

Diseases Typical to Orange Ray subjects: Chronic Asthma, Phlegmatic Fevers, Bronchitis, Wet Cough, Gout, Chronic Rheumatism.

Diseases readily cured by the use of Orange; The foregoing, and Inflammation of the Kidneys, Gall Stones, Prolapsus, Cessation of Menstruation (Fem.), Mental Debility, Epilepsy, Cholera, etc.

Characteristics of Orange: Orange has a freeing action upon bodily and mental functions, relieving repressions; it combines physical energy with mental wisdom, inducing transmutation between the lower nature and the higher; it outweans moronic tendencies helping to unfold and raise the mentality—it is therefore often termed the "Wisdom Ray". By its use we are able to heal the physical body and at the same time inculcate into the mind some understanding of how the body may be kept in good repair once it is healed. Orange is warming, cheering, non-electric, non-stringent.

Locality and Affinity: Orange controls the Second Chakram, or Splenic Centre (and Pancreas), assisting in the assimilative, distributive and circulatory processes. It holds the key-vibration to the doorway of the spleen. Through its active rays the essences of all foods are assimilated, classified, and distributed to the various creative centres, or departments, of the human system.

The effect of Orange upon the mentality is to aid the assimilation of new ideas, to induce mental enlightenment with a sense of freedom from limitations. Excess of orange on the mind and emotions, in some instances, may incline to over-indulgence, so it should always be used discriminately, realizing that we must ever prescribe Colour with Awareness of our individual uniqueness—no two persons, even when identical Ray types, reacting in exactly the same way. No two treatments, therefore, should ever be precisely alike, the individual factors of the subject's Ray, his colours of Inspiration, Activity and Rest[1] always varying the basic prescription.

Orange Rays, as well as their complementary Blue rays, are used for certain, yet quite diverse, mental disorders. Some of us are supernormal in our excitability, while others are phlegmatically subnormal.

A wise man once said that all men are queer in one way or another. Paramhansa Yogananda put a gentle smile into serious words when he remarked that we are all somewhat crazy, but that the great thing was patiently to try to understand each other's craziness, and learn from each. Only in this way do we gain wider tolerance, and expansion of the Heart-Force.

"When," says Ivah Bergh Whitten, "you put aside that self-adjustable tape-line, and realize that were you that other person you are about to condemn, or of his Ray type, you would have reactions and impulses similar to his." Therefore silence criticism into tolerance and Wisdom.

The Orange Light (Orangelume) helps to induce this tolerance. At the same time it strengthens the Will. For this reason it is used to supply egoic stimulus to those suffering from mental debility.

Mental Debility is often a form of mental paralysis—an inability to cope with Life's trials. New courage, firmer Will-power and stability are needed. Orange supplies it.

To this end we have prepared for such cases, at times, special Orange-radiating lamps. These are either spherical or egg-shaped and radiate a powerful, uplifting and bucyant vibration. Such treatment should eventually be followed by submersion in the subject's own Ray colour (further individualized by his colour of Inspiration), the Ray tone being the greatest general tonic an individual can receive.

Transmutation of the sexual forces is accomplished on the Orange Ray. At times of such excitement it is greatly helpful to visualize an Orange light at the feet and pointing upward, breathing deeply in affirmation, raising the consciousness out

[1] "Using Colour," by Ivah B. Whitten, A.M.I.C.A. (in preparation).

of physical desires and repressions, and liberating the energy up into the spine to the brain for greater creative attainments.

Diseases usually grouped as physical complaints may be treated successfully with Orange as follows:

Prolapsus: Position the subject so that legs and feet are raised slightly above the trunk level, at an angle of about 45 degrees above horizontal. In cases of emergency obtain a kitchen chair, tilt it over on to the floor so that, with the four feet off the ground, the back makes an angle with the floor of about half-a-right-angle. Then rest the patient's legs up the chair back, focusing Orangelume at the knees directed trunkwards. Try to obtain the subject's co-operation with easy "upward" Orange breathing, lifting the consciousness, circulation, bodily functions, and organs, *upward*.

Treatment twice daily will soon cause the organs to re-adjust themselves properly.

Chronic Asthma: It is noteworthy that persons with deep broad chests are seldom prone to this disease—it is essentially a complaint of shallow breathers.

Shallow breathing denotes either fear, too much intro-version, sense of futility, or lack of creative interest or purpose in life—or just laziness.

Asthma, there is much evidence to believe, originates from living *fear*fully instead of *power*fully. Once the deep breathing power-consciousness of the ego asserts itself, Asthma departs with all its cramping, hindering limitations.

The disease is augmented, outwardly, by contractive, humid atmospheres, and continued dampness. After all, these are but the physical counterparts of similar mental atmospheres.

It should always be remembered that the lungs are great energizing organs, and the throat itself has been termed, by metaphysicians, one of the greatest creative and power centres in the entire body. If we would have dynamic health in them, we must charge them with the cosmic breath. These are things of the spirit. (Nevertheless, the Ego-lux has helped many consciously to breathe away the origin of Asthma.)

Practise the Orange colour-breathing affirmation, breath-ing not only from the lungs but from the pit of the stomach also—feel as though you are breathing from your very feet. Do not breathe through the mouth, for the sudden impact of cold or damp air as it reaches the throat cannot help but be detrimental. In breathing through the nostrils every provision has been made, so that air is more acceptable as it reaches the chest and lungs.

Deep, easy rhythmical breathing is necessary in order to keep the blood in proper circulation and free from poisons and mucous.

In most cases the digestive organs are impaired at first and the whole system loses the healthy tone of vigour and strength, and then phlegm increases in the system and heat decreases. The cough is dried up by cold in the lungs and nature resorts to hurried breathing to remove phlegm.

Orangegas, to reinforce Orange affirmative breathing, will be found excellent as an animating force for the blood, to clear away those bad early morning conditions.

Orangero and Orangelume should complete the cure.

A dose of half-a-medicine-glassful of Orangero, with the chill taken off by the sun, should be taken every ten minutes for an hour, and Orangelume should be focused on the chest and throat. The patient is sure to feel some relief within this period.

The treatment of Orangegas, Orangero and Orangelume should be repeated after three to four hours, if necessary, until the severity of the condition is entirely broken up. During healthy intervals eat plentifully of oranges, or take one ounce of Orangero in between meals.

Many cases suffering from prolonged intense chronic bronchial asthma have found immediate relief after taking Orange treatment.

After the chronic symptoms have been finally dispersed, the treatment may be concluded with Cerulume upon the throat, to tone up the laryngeal power centre to its true health vibration.

It has been found that some persons get relief from Blue-Indigo water and light treatment (Indigolo and Indigolume), but that is always at the early stages of the complaint when it has not become chronic. Such persons are generally Red or Orange Ray subjects (*i.e.* those having reddish colour predominant in their systems) who expose themselves to cold.

Gall Stones: Observance of a number of cases of this disease lead to the conviction that there is usually an underlying mental-emotional origin to this trouble. Wherever a bitter resentment has crystallized in the mind and been persisted in without the divine solvent of love, the gall of bitterness tends to precipitate and crystallize in the bladder.

First steps towards dissolving these sharp, ragged crystals is to breathe in, and circulate within, the Peachy Universal Love rays—the Divine solvent. Start inhaling in the early morning to smoothen the attitude to life and to the people who "grate" on you. Refuse to be bitterly harsh or emotionally upset. Then introduce Orangero and Orangelume. One case of gall-stones coupled with rheumatism in the lower limbs was treated in the following manner: The patient relaxed on a couch face-downward. Magnetic hand-sweeps from the hollow of the back downwards on the legs and feet were first employed, eliminatingly. Then Orangelume was focused on the feet for ten minutes. Twenty minutes were then spent raising the Orangelume up the back of the legs and lower spine till the lumbar vertebra was reached.

The Orangelume was focused for some fifteen minutes on this Splenic centre and circular etheric massage was given with outward freeing sweeps. The patient had six treatments.

When shortly afterward, she had medical and X-rays examination, she was reported free from gall crystals and the rheumatic symptoms had vanished.

To prevent the possibility of any recurrence of this disease it is essential to remove the bitter crystals entirely from the mental-emotional nature.

Inflammation of the Kidneys: If caused by gravel, the Orangelume will remove it as well as the gravel. Cures of longstanding disease have come to our attention. One case suffered from occasional attacks for seven years, when he was advised to use Orangelume on the kidneys, and to take Orangero internally. On the third day he passed a large quantity of small gravel and since then he was permanently cured of kidney pains.

Bronchitis: Chronic cases show a low state of health and require Orange treatment for some months, slow treatment being best. The patient may not feel much better for a week or two, but as soon as the Orange colour has put the stomach and bowels in order, the disease begins to disappear by degrees.

Wet Cough: *i.e.* the type in which thick phlegm is readily thrown out of the system, is cured by Orange treatment;

Orangero being taken internally and Orangelume upon the lungs will put the chest into a healthy condition. The production of phlegm in the system is arrested and the existing phlegm expelled. Slow treatment is necessary; two doses in the morning and one in the evening will suffice to cure the disease in a fortnight's time.

Epilepsy, or Falling Sickness: This disease is generally due to a series of continued shocks inducing a constant state of fear in the mind which arrest the inflow of life-currents into the finer bodies. The result is the devitalization of the nerves and bodily functions. Orangero for internal use would tone the whole system and Cerulume for the head would poise the brain to withstand sudden attacks. The treatment should be continued for a fortnight without interruption, whether there be any attacks of epilepsy or not during that period.

Paralysis: The transmuting Orange rays cure states of paralysis which are due to emotional reactions. (See Red section for method and procedure.)

Cholera: Jwala Prasada, the Indian Colour Healer, has cured Cholera with Orange treatment when the life-force had been reduced to a very low ebb. But in the incipient stages he has found that Blue has effected the most certain cures. (See Blue Ray section, page 86).

Diseases to which those on the Orange Ray in general are prone are very closely related to those inhering to the Yellow with which Orange merges. We will therefore consider the Yellow Ray next.

HEALING COLOUR-BREATHING AFFIRMATION
YELLOW RAY

O Yellow beams of Gold
Enrichen my Intelligence;
O Strengthen thy Sun-radiance,
Aged-Wisdom in Youth unfold.

. .

Empower my Solar Plexus
To digest, assimilate,
Inhaling Golden Atoms
Of Joy—all Fear Abate.

. , .

O Saffron Rays of Wisdom Prana,
Flow in Golden Currency,
Feeding cells with Cosmic Manna,
Throughout my Entirety.

When you get up in the morning, stand in front of the open window, sufficiently clad, and take about twenty deep breaths, slowly in and slowly out.

As you breathe, try to visualize the Sun-radiant Air as enriching the Earth—the Golden Currents within the Earth and all its inhabitants.

See this flood of Yellow Light flowing into your body, permeating it, and enlightening every particle of it.

Then go ahead with your specific treatment, or with your day's work. Before long you will notice a surprising improvement in the circulation of your affairs; in your everyday life and circumstances, not alone mentally but materially as well.

Test this out for yourself. Don't do it hurriedly or with the expectation of quick results. Do it conscientiously and sensibly.

Chapter VII

YELLOW

METALS radiating Yellow: Gold, Barium, Calcium, Chromium, Nickel, Zinc, Copper, Strontium, Cadmium, Cobalt. Manganese, Aluminium, Titanium.

Chemicals, Elements and Gases: Carbon, Sodium, Phosphorus, and many alkalines.

The best glass to use in treatment contains Iron compounds in tne presence of Manganese, Uranium or Red Lead oxides, and Sulphur.

Foods: Parsnips, Yellow Peppers, Golden Corn, Yams, Banana Squash, Marrow, Pineapples, Bananas, Lemons, Grapefruit, Honey-dew Melons, and most yellow-skinned fruits and vegetables.

Typical Diseases to which Yellow Ray subjects are prone: Stomach troubles, Indigestion, and the variety of complaints related thereto: Constipation, Flatulence, Liver troubles, Diabetes, Blind Piles, Eczema and skin troubles, Leprosy, Nervous Exhaustion.

Characteristics and Effects of Yellow: These Rays carry positive magnetic currents and are non-stringent, having an alkalising effect which strengthens the nerves. Yellow Rays are awakening, inspiring and vitally stimulating to the higher mentality—the reasoning faculties—upon which they have a very powerful and remarkable effect. Through enlightenment, Yellow thus aids self-control.

Locality and Affinity: Yellow stimulates the Third Chakram, or Solar Plexus, the great brain of the nervous system, controlling the digestive processes in the stomach and brain. Yellow helps to purify the system through its eliminative action on the liver and intestines; it cleanses the billions of bodily pores which expel and impel; it improves the texture of the skin, healing scars and other blemishes. Yellow also has an *enriching* effect upon the intellectual departments of the brain. The exoteric interpretation of Yellow as Fear is grossly incorrect. Certainly Fear apprehended in the brain is often *felt* in the Solar Plexus because of the very negation of the positivizing rays of Yellow. The colour of Fear is basically Gray, although mustardy tints are sometimes seen in that Gray.

Yellow represents a material to which has been accorded the highest human value—Gold. When we wish to appreciate the value of a thing we customarily compare it with gold—"Worth its weight in gold" is a common remark regarding that which we highly prize. In conferring highest honours or rewards we bestow gold medals, gold watches, gold cups, and gold purses.

The golden crown on the Head controlling the State, symbolically represents the superiority of Heaven over the Earthly kingdom. This suggests the spiritual quality of Gold (the Zenith of transmuted metals) and of the Yellow Ray, reflected by painters in depicting saints or spiritual teachers with a golden halo around their heads—the seal of Wisdom.

Solomon, according to the Biblical story, when asked to choose amongst many good things, chose Wisdom. "He did not," comments Dr. Hylton, "ask for material gold—that had already circulated to him, he wisely chose the magnetic spiritual counterpart, Wisdom," so that he might thereby be enabled to make the best use of the Yellow Ray in both its aspects; in the aspect of Knowledge, and in the wise administration of its material counterpart.

Wisdom is to the mind, much as gold is to the material. Just as the usefulness of Gold in the world's body lies first in acquisition and then in currency (*i.e.* distribution), so also the Golden Rays in the human body play their most important parts in the acquisitive and circulative departments or functions.

Those who incarnate on the Yellow Ray have a searching desire to acquire knowledge and Wisdom. Their troubles usually lie in the gathering in of more than they can readily digest and put into circulation, both mentally and physically.

Is it not vitally interesting to note the types of diseases to which Yellow Ray subjects are largely prone: Stomach, Liver, Digestive troubles and Diabetes (all assimilative complaints), then Constipation, Diarrhœa, Eczema, and other skin diseases (all circulative complaints). With this understanding we have the key to their cure.

People born on this Ray are usually more active mentally than physically, in fact they have a tendency to neglect, ignore or disdain, the physical body, asserting the superiority of the Mind. We find them living "sitting" lives, or in sedentary occupations, inducive to eliminative and circulative troubles. With these points in mind let us proceed to their cure.

Dyspepsia: There are two causes of dyspepsia—the increase of Red in the system or the increase of Blue, depending respectively upon whether the subject has incarnated at the Blue end of the spectrum or at the Red.

In persons who suffer from an increase of Red colour, the constitution is generally lean and emaciated; whilst those who suffer from increase of Blue are generally fat.

The increase of Blue is indicated by stoutness. This is usually caused by want of exercise, sedentary life or occupation, resulting in poor circulation.

Affirmative Yellow breathing should be commenced early in the mornings and Ambergas taken at noon on bright days. Half-a-medicine-glassful of Ambero should be taken frequently between meals. Amberlume should be focused on the Solar Plexus for thirty minutes at a time, daily. In about a week's time improvement will be evident.

The increase of Red can be toned down by the use of Indigogas, Indigolo and Indigolume. These taken into the system cool down the irritation of the stomach and bring about proper digestion. But this disease, if of long standing, requires slow treatment.

Colour gas, water and light treatment should be given twice daily and continued for one or two months consecutively and the disease will then disappear completely.

Diabetes: In this chronic complaint the patient originally suffers from want of proper digestion. More fat is formed in the system than blood. Ambero taken internally, and Amberlume focused on the Solar Plexus, twice daily, will decrease the formation of fat, and increase the blood in the system. Constipation, which is very often an unavoidable consequence of this disease would then be removed.

Two months treatment is necessary completely to check the formation of fat as well as for the increase of blood supply in the system. Thirst will decrease as the fat is decreased. Of course, long and continuous treatment is necessary in the case of such slow and devitalizing diseases.

Heartburn and Waterbrash are signs of indigestion. They are generally found in phlegmatic temperaments and can be cured by an ounce of Ambero. These sensations will then cease and proper digestive functions will commence.

Flatulence in Stomach and Bowels (also usually, the result of improper digestion although it can have hidden origins in some cases), may be cured by a medicine-glassful of Ambero, between meals, *sipped slowly*. When it occurs on an empty stomach, it is also cured by Ambero, and Ambergas, if accompanied by feverish conditions Ceruleo and Cerulegas should be used first, and taken repeatedly every three hours.

Piles are caused by a static attitude to Life, or by sedentary habits, habitual constipation, pregnancy, excessive horse-back-riding but lack of other free exercise, also free indulgence of stimulating drinks, and highly seasoned foods, etc., can bring on this complaint.

Blind Piles can be cured by Ambero taken internally, thus removing the constipation and reducing the severity of the disease. External application of Ceruleo and Cerulume remove inflammation of the piles and contract same.

Yellow should not be used for bleeding-piles; instead, the astringent external Blue treatment will bring the safest relief.

Constipation: Ambero and Amberlume, in homeopathic doses, offer the perfect stimulant to excite sluggish bowels, and a slow, steady use of this colour is sure to cure constipation no matter however longstanding it may be. Help the circulative rhythm of the body-functions by deep Yellow breathing, and take Ambero in between meals as frequently as the need be. Thirty minutes morning and evening with the Amberlume focused on the navel will prove a great aid.

Should too much Yellow be taken at any one time, with over-laxative effect, it is well to remember that a dose of the complementary Ceruleo will restore the necessary balance.

Paralysis: In our treatise on the Red Ray we dealt with the energizing value of Red in certain cases of paralysis of the lower limbs. It should always be remembered that this is primarily a disease of the brain and nerves, which control the limbs, therefore Yellow is often greatly helpful in obtaining the desired release and control. As already pointed out, Paralysis is basically a lack of self-control, the inability to order the nerve-force into circulation and activity. "Paralysis," says Dr. Edwin Babbitt, "forms one of the diseases of the nerves inasmuch as the particular disease hits either upon the electrical or the thermal nerve.

"Though caused largely in the motor region of the cerebrum, it is also caused by the condition of the spine or the nerves themselves. A pressure of the blood upon the motor region of the right brain will usually cause a left hemiplegia. Paraplegia, or paralysis of both sides, more commonly affects both legs and hips and usually comes from a lesion of both sides of the spinal column. Electricity from the battery and static machine have helped some cases, but the greater power to reach the nerves must come from the more refined elements of sunlight, especially the Yellow Ray. Amberlume over the occiput and cervix for hemiplegia, or over the lumbar, and sacral region, for paraplegia would be fine, and if followed by truly magnetic massage with many down-strokes for motor-paralysis, and up-strokes for sensory paralysis, would be doubly good."

"Yellow," says Jwala Prasada, the Indian colour-therapist, "is an effective treatment for all kinds of leprosy, but the cure takes six months to be complete. Two doses daily are sufficient, one in the morning and one at sunset, or a little before. This should be continued for a week or ten days until the bowels are regularly open, the bad matter being discharged out of the system in small quantities.

"The patient after a month has more blood in the system than before. In three months' time, blood will ooze out of the wounds instead of watery substance, and in six months' time all wounds will have become cured. In two months more the system will be quite renovated and there need be no fear of recurrence of this disease.

"Rice, milk, fish, curd, cheese and raw sugar should be avoided during the treatment, and also salt, for this assists in producing bad water in the system." Gram is the best food with a little of wheat in it. Butter is necessary for the system to meet the large demand for nourishment and renovation.

Healing Colour-Breathing Affirmation
GREEN RAY

O Ray of Emerald Sympathy
Sustain, upbuild my wayward Heart:
Its strings attune in Symphony,
Teach me to do my poiseful part.

. . .

O Chlorophyllic builder, true—
Heart-force in fields and men renew;
From Thee the tempo true is bidden
O Strengthen Thou the beat, the Rhythm.

. . .

The pulse of Brotherhood regain;
Bring forth the honey, harboured, hidden,
In human hearts now freely given,
Sweet food in All, for all, sustain!

Drink in the delight of early morning rays, shimmering from the dewy bejewelled grass; and O the refreshment of green foliage after rain! Visualize the sunshine sparkling from the shining trees at noon; and lastly, the glancing dusk-rays dancing through the leaves. Here is Nature's Emerald, flashing Prana!

Drink deeply of these verdant rays, poised between the Gold of Wisdom and the Blue of Heaven!

Chapter VIII

GREEN

METALS radiating Green: Sodium, Copper, Nickel, Chromium, Cobalt, Platinum, Aluminium, Titanium.

Chemicals, Elements, Gases: Carbon, Nitrogen, Ferrous Sulphate, Hydrochloric Acid, Chlorophyll.

The best glass to use contains combines of the above metals and chemicals; and iron-oxide.

Foods: Most green vegetables and fruits that are neither acidulous or alkaline in reaction.

Typical Diseases to which Green Ray subjects are prone: Heart troubles, Blood-Pressure, Ulcers, Cancer. The Green Ray is also invaluable for alleviating Headaches, Neuralgia, Influenza; Syphilis, Erysipelas.

Characteristics and effects of Green: Green is the colour of Nature, the colour of balanced strength, the colour of progress in mind and body. Green stands for harmony, possessing a soothing influence upon the nervous system. Hence the deep meaning of those beautiful words in the 23rd Psalm: "He maketh me to lie down in green pastures . . . beside the still waters," *i.e.* inhabit the planet Earth. Indian philosophy associates green with the waters of the Earth, maintaining that it increases the harmonic vibrations of our thoughts and brings peace to our senses. The desire for green fields and trees, after spells midst the city's grey stone and red brick, is the instinctive physical craving for Nature's colour tonic which soothes and restores. Green is neutral, at the fulcrum of the solar spectrum—the balancing point.

Green is neither heating nor stringent; neither acid nor alkaline. Apple-green is the radiance of Brotherhood—the vibration of impersonal motive, the common denominator in all Nature.

Locality and Affinity: Green stimulates the Cardiac Chakram, or Heart centre. Just as at the Heart of Nature we find the stimulus of green, so at the heart of the human system we find it also.

This colour affects our blood pressure in an unusual manner—the Yellow in it forces the brain to act more energetically and refreshingly, whilst the Blue half inculcates moderation of that pressure—an action very much like the tides; whereas with Red, which also increases the blood circulation, it does so more often through sudden emotional activity rather than through balanced mind activity.

It is interesting to note that our scientists and chemists now produce concentrates of this green essence of Nature, known as Chlorophyll, to stimulate and sustain the heart action. Such tablets are but densified light-waves. Verdilume, however, offers the finest medium for taking this sun-energy, which is thus one stage nearer its source.

When the Spring comes to the world, we are aware of the change by the coming of the green shoots from the trunks and limbs of trees and of green sprouts from the heart of seeds. We are accustomed to associate Spring with *new energy* in our own trunks, limbs, and hearts. After drab, colourless winter days we feel fresher and brighter within, brighter in spirit and better in health. Although we do not realize it, this is the action of the Green Ray of renewal upon our material and finer bodies which causes us to have these feelings.

Why do we send invalids "down to the country" to convalesce, despite better medical attention available in the cities? The fact is, we obtain actual material strength from the proximity of the expanse of greenery. It is an actual tonic to body, mind and spirit. It should be recalled that Yellow is the colour of Wisdom (Mind), Blue the colour of Truth (Spirit), and Green is the combination of Yellow and Blue offering a balanced body for both. It is because it is a tonic to the three main vehicles of the human-being that it is so successful a medicine.

Heart Troubles: These often originate at emotional levels, coming from an inversion, or bottling up of the Love Ray.

Many dear old maiden ladies suffer from this complaint because they have never found the natural expression for the fulness of their love. As the years have gone by they have withdrawn from any exhibition of their love lest they receive hurt from lack of response. Sometimes, secret jealousy or bitterness creeps into their souls, and the unpleasant mustardy shades of Green outpicture from their auras.

On the other hand, those with sweeter dispositions confine themselves to the love of pets, or to the love of flowers and gardens, which, though still involving a repressed love do afford outlets for the heart-force. It is lifetime full of such repressions that often causes Blood Pressure. Yet in the outlet of a garden—their little world,—there lies the secret of release, for soothing Soft Green is the antidote.

If the more humanly attuned Peachy Universal Love Breathing Affirmation does not come easily, then use the complementary Green Breathing Affirmation, realizing at-one-ment with the pulsating, compassionate, heart of *all* life on this Planet; so that your horizon extends far beyond the confines of your personal, mental and emotional being, as boundless as the Universe itself. Expand the little self into the larger, acknowledging kinship or Brotherhood, with all human, animal, plant and mineral Life. If you will, extend the confines of your garden to embrace the entire earth and all its inhabitants, with you serenely at its heart. In you the Emerald Life-Prana shines and flows, absorbing nature's chlorophyll stimulatingly. Share it generously with all.

The best times to do this are soon after sunrise, at noon, and at sunset. Then take Verdilume treatment, continuing the affirmation and colour breathing.

If suffering from low blood-pressure, focus the deep Verdilume over the heart for thirty minutes at a time, and breathe in the radiant energy. Between meals, at hourly intervals, drink half-a-glassful of Verdigo. Should high blood-pressure be the complaint, use light Verdilume instead of the deeper shade. Eat freely of green salad.

Neuralgic Headaches: Verdilume is the best treatment for such complaints. The colour soothes the heart and so adjusts the nerves of the sympathetic system and brain, that great relief is felt even by looking at this green light. People exhausted from tiresome nerve-spent days can be refreshened, in an hour or so, by sitting in Verdilume; such treatments produce strengthened and more optimistic trends of thought. When insomnia, lack of rest and relaxation are the sources of the complaint, treatment may be helpfully keyed to Indigo-Violet.

Transparent coloured celastoid eye-shades can prove very useful in this connection.

Ulcers: Verdilume will cure ulcers, though treatment will take a long time. Dr. Crile, the famous physician of Cleveland, recently told the Michigan Medical Association "that in his opinion peptic ulcers are caused by the discharge of electric batteries in the stomach. Fear may produce such disease, and faith may cure it. Anger tears down the body; love builds it up. Criticism and antagonism lessen personal capacities; commendation and admiration expand and enlarge them." Dr. Edwin Babbitt, and Jwala Prasada, both famous colour healers in their time, healed ulcers with the compassionate use of Green.

Syphilis is another perversion of the Love-force. Verdigo will cure any description of this disease; Verdilume should also be applied externally.

Erysipelas: Verdilume applied at the first symptoms, and thereafter, will prevent the malady going deeply into the system. This disease can begin very dangerously with an increase of heat and a tendency to ulceration, but cure can be readily effected with the timely use of the Green Ray.

Colds in the Head: Verdigo and Verdilume take away the bad effects of cold. Chronic cases have been cured very easily by this treatment, sometimes with the help of Indigo.

Mucous Fevers, Influenza, Whooping Cough and Croup are curable with Verdilume and Cerulume.

Influenza requires both Verdilume and Verdigo.

Boils if running, can be very soon cured by the application of Verdilume and Indigolume. Indigolume first draws out all the bad matter in the wound, and when it has done so, Verdilume sorks to turn pus into flesh and cures the wound by producing a healthy skin over it.

Carcinoma Mammæ: In the appendix to his valuable book Dr. C. E. Iredell gives several cases instancing the treatment of growths with Verdilume, all with conclusive results. He also employed other spectrum radiation in the treatment of this disease according to the location and condition.

Green, the great harmonizer, holding the balance in the spectrum, and in our lives, is a wonderful agent for neutralizing the inharmonious vibrations of malignant growths, and in tuning up the nervous system—thus imparting the *consciousness* of harmony and so reaching cause.

Cancer: This often originates through cruelty—a perversion of the love-force, either in this life-time, or in a past life. The Green Ray has a very important part to play in the treatment of this dread disease for which allopathy has no proper or effective medicine. Its alleviation should start with a change of consciousness, and by using the Universal and then the Green Ray Breathing Affirmation. Physical treatment may then follow with the administration of Verdigo internally, and by projecting Verdilume over the cancer externally. It has been found that Verdilume focused upon a compress of Yellow silk which has been soaked in brine, gives forth a highly refined or etheric radioactivity which corrects cancerous growths, but unlike regular radium treatment, it does not injure the surrounding normal tissue. Ivah Bergh Whitten, A.M.I.C.A., has produced a special colour technique for localized treatment of this world-wide scourge.[1]

[1] See "Colour and Cancer", by C. E. Iredell, M.D., M.R.C.P.
(out of print)

Healing Colour-Breathing Affirmation

BLUE RAY

O Tranquil Ray of Sapphire Blue,
Calm Thou my Mind in solace new,
In solace new;
Quench Thou all Fevers,
In Coolness new, as refreshing dew;
Tone Thou my Speech, O Ray of Blue—
And make It true,
And make It true;
Help me to learn, O Ray of Blue—
To Rest in You,
To Rest in You;
Help me to learn, O Ray of Blue—
To Speak anew,
To Speak anew;
Help me to learn, O Ray of Blue—
To Sing in You,
To Sing in You.

Imagine the Blue bright sky of an early summer morning—not a cloud on the horizon. Visualize yourself drinking in this shining Blue not only with your lungs but with every eager pore in your body.

Picture yourself, if you will, a skylark blithely aloft in summer's Blue expanse, trouble free.

Or perhaps you have flown high in an aeroplane, the Earth below seeming so small, unimportant, and far off; the Blue sky so expansive and all-embracing, so that for a while your entire consciousness and activity is bound up with It alone?

Try to recapture, or to visualize, that feeling when breathing in the Heavenly Blue.

Chapter IX

BLUE

METALS radiating Blue: Tin, Lead, Cobalt, Copper, Nickel, Zinc, Cadmium, Manganese, Aluminium, Titanium.

Chemicals, Elements, Gases: Copper Sulphate, Phosphoric Acid, Chloroform, Tannic Acid; Oxygen.

The best glass to use in the treatment of disease contains Oxides of Copper, and Ammonium Sulphate.

Foods: Most Blue Fruits, Blue Plums, Bilberries, etc. See "Colour and Diet" for fuller classification.

Typical Diseases to which Blue Ray subjects are prone: All Throat troubles; Laryngitis, Goitre, Sore-throat, Hoarseness; Teething; also the following diseases can be cured by Blue: Fevers; Scarlet Fever, Typhoid, Cholera, Bubonic Plague, Smallpox, Chickenpox, Measles, Aphthæ, Apoplexy, Hysteria, Epilepsy, Palpitation, Spasms; Acute Rheumatism; then again, Vomiting, Purging, Thirst, Dysentery, Diarrhœa, Jaundice, Biliousness, Colic; also Inflamed Bowels, Inflamed Eyes, Stings, Itches, Toothache; Headaches, Nervous Disorders, Insomnia, Painful Menstruation, Shock, etc.

Characteristics and effects of Blue: "The Blue Ray is one of the greatest antiseptics in the world," claimed Dr. Edwin Babbitt. Its light is cooling, electric, soporific, astringent. Blue light transmitted through the correct glass compounds will stop bleeding of the lungs, decrease fevers, cure sore throat and do many other seemingly incomprehensible things, if properly applied. The Blue Ray bears upon every facet of Truth; Science and Invention exhibit this aspect of the Blue Ray's influence. It would appear to have its negative side, such as applying inventive research to gain physical advantages, e.g. producing new weapons of war. Also to "feel blue" indicates the instinctive recognition of this sedative property of the Blue Ray. Nevertheless, Blue has its positive side ascribable to the things of the Spirit: Truth, Loyalty, Reliability—hence we speak of "Blue as Heavens", "True Blue", and of being "Blue-Blooded".

It has been said that Truth is all-conquering, and somewhat merciless, although this is more apparent than actual. Have you ever tried to live, say, for one day in an atmosphere of perfect truth? If you would realize the exact truth in all

things, then you would be perfect tune with the Blue Ray
and its calm serenity would be of great benefit. Blue is only
fully used in a state of perfection.

Locality and Affinity of Blue: Blue controls the Laryngeal
Chakram, or Throat Centre, often referred to as the Power
Centre and "the greatest creative centre in man's body".
This is because it is his greatest centre of sxlf-expression—in
speech. How well we might often meditate on the creative,
or destructive power of speech! Relaxing, soothing, Blue rays
will also bring great calm and peace to the mind that is
worried, excited, or in constant nervous state.

Before treating for any specific complaint the patient
should try to universalize his consciousness, and then visualize
himself as flooded with the Blue light—breathing it in and
sending it to the affected part.

Laryngitis, or Inflammation of the Larynx should be
treated with half-a-glassful of Ceruleo every half an hour.
Gargle with some of it. Supplement this with regular
Cerulume treatment focused upon the throat.

I recall the case of a well-known North of England clergyman who had the embarrassing experience of losing his voice
in the middle of an important address. The minister was
finally obliged to cease speaking entirely, and he asked his
congregation to join with him in silent prayer, in which he
asked for strength to continue and make the culminating
points of his message. Almost immediately, he found himself
in strong, vibrant voice again. Afterwards more than one
psychically developed member of his audience came to him
and declared they had seen a bright Blue light surrounding
his throat, when he had made his plea in mid-address. The
clergyman who mentioned this to me has since adopted a
focused Blue light successfully to remedy this "voice-
disappearing" tendency.

Another case of loss of voice which has unique points of
interest was treated by Ivah B. Whitten, by "proxy" through
a student at the time visiting in Lake Worth, Florida. "A
woman was being driven by her husband to give a recital.
Arriving at the auditorium, she got out on the kerbside
whilst her husband commenced to get out from behind the
wheel on the opposite or road side. Suddenly, she saw a
drunken driver zig-zagging madly down the street, but before
she could speak to warn her husband, the drunken driver

swerved and pinned him between the cars, killing him instantly.

"When the wife tried to speak her vocal cords would not function. For several days she was dumb. Then her speaking voice returned, but she could not sing a note. It was at this stage that she went south for the winter, as did my pupil who had just finished the initial lessons in Colour Awareness, and was an enthusiastic follower of Colour. She wrote for advice and I had one of the colour lamps shipped to her. The woman was kept in the Blue light (Cerulume) by means of cellophane over the windows, and the Blue light from the lamp was focused on the throat for forty minutes twice each day, followed by Violet (Violume) super-imposed by Blue, which was applied for one hour.

"Then one day, while under treatment, she sang again. A week later she regained her former singing voice-control, which occurred nine weeks from the date of starting treatment and before finishing her course in Colour Awareness which she had been studying along with the treatments.

"I have always considered it significant that at the 9th Lesson which deals with the Throat Centre she should have recovered, and that she herself was incarnated on the 5th or Blue Ray, treated in that lesson."

The case comes to hand of a young lady who was taken so severely with laryngitis, with also some irritation of the lungs, that she had to abandon the school in which she was teaching, and go home. She was advised to take a Blue chromo-jar and to leave the top off, place her hand over the opening to shut in the air, and after the sun had shone into it for three or four seconds, to put her mouth and nose to the opening and take one long inhalation. This inhalation of Cerulegas was to be repeated at least twenty times. It was reported that the treatment acted like magic so that the next day she went to work in good condition.

Hoarseness: This is best treated with Cerule in small, yet frequent doses. Start the day with the Blue Breathing Affirmation and exercise, and then focus Cerulume on the throat for half an hour. Take half a glassful of Ceruleo three times in the morning, and again three times in the afternoon; use a little also gently to gargle, holding the water at the back of the mouth to tone the throat.

Sore Throat: This disease is generally caused by cold or exposure. It is indicated by difficulty in swallowing, the throat often being reddened and swollen. It sometimes becomes dangerous when inflammation increases rapidly.

It is very easily cured by gargling with Ceruleo repeated at intervals of three hours. The complaint should pass within twenty-four hours, or at the lengthiest forty-eight hours. Chronic cases have been cured in about four or five days' time.

Ceruleo is thus good for all throat diseases which generally are caused by an accumulation of heat for which Blue is the specific antidote. It acts like a charm.

Aphthæ, or Speckled Thrush: Small white specks on the tongue, lips, cheeks, gums and on other parts on the inside of the mouth, usually of infants. Sometimes the disease descends to the stomach and bowels, and then it becomes dangerous. It is due to increase of heat, and restlessness is often observed, accompanied with fever. The simple treatment for this disease is Ceruleo, or better still Cerulelac given in very small quantities, say a quarter of a glassful, or even less, every half hour, for three or four hours; then allow Nature to work out the cure for some hours. After twenty-four hours the treatment may be recommenced if the disease is not quite cured.

Dentition or Teething: Young infants naturally suffer from this a great deal, and weak children often cannot overcome it. Heat is engendered by the complaint sometimes affecting the eyes, and then the infant feels the worst, for it cannot open its eyes and granulations are formed. The simple method to cure this disease is with Cerulume. The infant should be kept in it for some hours every day until the heat subsides. Ceruleo may be used advantageously with discrimination, but it is unwise to try to use water inwardly when Cerulume is quite sufficient to cure. Many infants die from this, and it would be well if parents would use this simple method of cure.

Inflammation of the brain: Cerulume is the best treatment for this disease, found amongst children, it begins with fever and restlessness, and should unconsciousness eventuate it is likely to prove serious. Nevertheless, Cerulume administered even at late stages of the disease will remove the urgent symptoms at once, and it is sure to cure the patient eventually.

Goitre: This disease has been cured by focusing Cerulume on to the subject's throat for periods of half to three-quarters of an hour, accompanied by gentle and also etheric massage. After each treatment the swelling has been reduced considerably, evidenced by the looseness of the outer skin. One case was treated once to twice a week only, and after some six weeks of steady improvement the goitre practically disappeared. Had treatments been possible more frequently, the goitre would undoubtedly have disappeared in much less time. A gargle frequently with Ceruleo would be a great help towards the quicker passing of this complaint.

Gumboil: This is caused by exposure to cold or through a decayed tooth. It may be cured readily by repeatedly filling the mouth with Ceruleo and keeping the gumboil immersed in it for some time. The heat will be decreased and the boil will subside.

Fevers: "This disease, varied in its character, claims the largest share in the mortality of human beings," says Jwala Prasada. In most cases the cause is the same, viz. the increase of red in the system. Sometimes it affects the brain, then it is called Brain Fever; sometimes it affects the bowels, then it is called Typhoid; at other times it affects the liver and then it is called Bilious Fever. On other occasions it affects the entire body through partial exposure and sudden changes of temperature, then it is termed Remittent Malarious Fever; and when the exposure is more severe it is called Intermittent Fever. Sometimes the constitution possesses bad matter and nature tries to throw it off,—the process employed by it is fever, whereby the matter is forced out of the body, as in the case of Smallpox, Scarlet Fever, Erysipelas. Then there are Mucous Fevers which dry up the mucous and are known as Influenza, Croup, Whooping Cough; there may be all manner of descriptions of them, but all are due to the undue increase of red colour, and the sole aim is to reduce the excess of that colour in the system.

Nature assists in the cure, to a great degree, carrying the remedy to the place where it is required. Thus, for instance, a man suffering from Dysentery, Ceruleo taken internally affects the bowels at such times more than any other body part. So it is not conclusive to treat the affected part directly only; if colour-solarized water is taken internally it will reach the diseased part and effect the cure. However, it is always better, when practicable, to throw the coloured light on the portion of the body affected by heat, for this is intended to bring about the cure all the sooner.

Typhus: This can be cured very readily with Cerulume alone. However, it is always better to administer Ceruleo which effects the loosening of the bowels.

Typhoid: This can be cured by Ceruleo alone; to avoid exposure, the stomach should always remain covered until complete cure is obtained.

Remittent and Intermittent Fevers: Ceruleo alone can affect cure, although in some severe cases where the temperature is extreme, Cerulume would also prove highly beneficial.

Malarial Fevers, however, are keyed to digestive troubles and require Yellow.

Eruptive Fevers: During these fevers no attempt should be made to check nature discharging unwanted matter from the system, but care should be taken to check the dangerous symptoms through the discriminate use of Colour.

Smallpox, Measles, Chickenpox, Erysipelas: If in any of these diseases there be great thirst, Ceruleo should be administered; when delirium commences, Cerulume would be beneficial; checking the symptoms in their progress is very dangerous and is likely to end fatally.

Cholera: Blue is the best remedy to cure Cholera; in the incipient stages, Jwala Prasada says, "There are many symptoms of this disease and I have found out by experience that any of such symptoms existing by itself has been cured by Blue Water (Ceruleo). I cure thirst by Blue water; I cure vomiting by Blue water; I stop purging by Blue water; I cure spasms by Blue water. Thus it is most probable and reasonable that Blue water will cure also when all symptoms combine in one system as in Cholera. The most urgent symptoms are removed first by two or three doses of Blue water, and the patient recovers in about six hours' time. Cholera is the sudden increase of Red in the system, and this heat reaches the very source of Life, the navel, where pranapan are knotted together to sustain life. By extraordinary heat this knot is at once loosened and both these Life currents are no longer controlled by each other and take their own course—the pran tries to go up and produces vomiting and nausea, and the apan tries to go down and produces purging. The pulse goes down at once for the Life point has been attacked by heat. It is yet to be experimented if a cold compress of Blue water (Ceruleo) on the navel, combined with a focused Blue light (Cerulume) thereon, can cure all the symptoms. Strong men who possess red colour in abundance are the most prone to the disease. Blue water also acts as a preventive." Meat and heating foods should be avoided, vegetable-and-fruit diet is strongly recommended.

Bubonic Plague: The importance of Blue as a saviour of life cannot be over-estimated. In Bombay thousands of lives have been saved from succumbing to Bubonic Plague, by administration of Ceruleo.

Dysentery: Ceruleo cures this disease in two days. Meat and starches should be avoided. Sago, Rice, Arrowroot, etc., are the best foods. Also Cerulelac (or milk kept in a blue bottle and solarized for ten minutes) would be a nourishment as well as a remedy.

Palpitation: This may also be cured with Ceruleo or Verdigo, taken internally.

Bilious attack: Ceruleo cures this complaint; three doses of it taken every two hours should remove the biliousness.

Diarrhœa: This can also be checked by the use of Ceruleo.

Colic: Ceruleo is the specific for these gripes. A dose of one ounce taken every ten minutes will cure the patient in about one hour. Three doses should be given and then nature allowed to complete the cure.

Bleeding Piles: External application of Ceruleo and Cerulume is sure to give relief.

Inflammation of the bowels: This is a dangerous disease but may readily be cured by Ceruleo, the doses being regulated by the exigencies of each case.

Jaundice: This is indicated by yellow skin, yellowishness in the eyes, and "yellow vision"; everything appears yellow to the jaundiced eye. Ceruleo and Indigolo cure this disease very quickly; the doses should be regulated according to the severity of the case.

Cuts, Bruises, Burns: All these may be remedied by using wet compresses of Ceruleo which takes away the burning sensation quickly and absorbs any heat in even less time. Blue is the perfect styptic and should be used in all cases of bleeding; the Red being contra-indicated.

Stings of all kinds: Ceruleo is the specific. It absorbs the

heat and relief is felt at once. When inflammation is evident
Cerulume on the inflamed part will check and reduce it.

Hydrophobia is attended by feverishness, great thirst, and
loss of appetite. Treat externally by administering Cerulume
to the wound for two or three hours daily and wash the
wound with Ceruleo, if possible keeping a wet compress of
Ceruleo thereon in between light treatment. Internally, take
one medicine-glassful of Ceruleo every three hours for the
first three days and when symptoms decrease follow with but
two to three doses daily, and after that just one dose upon
retiring.

Animals also respond readily to colour-treatment; Ceruleo
and Cerulelac will prevent them feeling the heat so greatly in
hot weather and have been known to antidote severe
poisoning.

The following Constitutional Diseases can be remedied
readily with Blue:

Acute Theumatism is curable by Cerulume and Ceruleo.
Chronic Rheumatism should be remedied by Orange (see
Orange Section).

Female Diseases: Certain troubles can be checked by the
use of Ceruleo taken internally. Doses should be regulated
according to the exigencies of the case.

The metaphysician has long known that Fear is the
directly traceable cause of all Pulmonary diseases; that to
eradicate Fear is to start a permanent cure.

Drawing in the Blue light of Poise and Serenity, and *fixing*
it by *Colour-Breathing* re-establishes the POWER-CON-
SCIOUSNESS which is so directly keyed to this Blue rate of
vibration. Then, if the case is of long standing, it is best to
disinfect with the deeper Indigolume in order to cast out the
atomic impurities discarded during the bombardment of
atoms. This bombardment of atoms by Cosmic forces is
constantly causing our entire atomic structure to split up and
multiply; within this process—stimulated as it is by Colour—
may be found the specific for complete cure.

It is within the radiance of this Blue-Indigo light that
much of this rebirth of cells constantly goes on, for within
our microcosm, our atoms never die, but split up into new
substances, new life expressions, and perpetual activity.

Healing Colour-Breathing Affirmation
INDIGO RAY

O Deep Rays, of Indigo Blue,
Bathe my Eyes, with tender hue—
Give me Sight, to see anew,
Give me Light, for seeing True.

. . .

O Deep Rays, of Indigo Blue,
Bathe my Ears, with deeper hue,
Tone my ears to hear anew—
Tune my Mind to hearing True.

. . .

O Deep Rays, of Indigo Blue,
Bring me in Devotion's hours,
The Balm, the Purity in Mental Showers—
Release new Fragrance from brain flowers,
Sweeping all brown leaves away.

In the Arizonan and Sahara Deserts, the high midnight sky is often clear Indigo. Stars stand out twice as real, the air more refreshing than man's best wine. Drink deeply of this enchanting Indigo!

Or, perhaps you have seen the scintillating Blauensee, the Blue Lake of Switzerland, at the foot of giant falls. This crystal lake, and the trout in it, are of bright deep Indigo.

Imagine yourself, if you will, one of these free trout drinking ever deeper of the rippling Indigo water and light, flowing in and over your entire body and mind.

Chapter X

INDIGO

METALS radiating Indigo: Chromium, Iron, Copper, Strontium, Titanium.

Chemicals: Potassium Bromide, Cupro-Diammonium Sulphate, Chloral Hydrate; Oxygen.

The best glass to use in treatment contains Cupro-Diammonium Sulphate, the main constituent of "Mazarine" glass.

Foods: Partake of both the Blue and the Violet.

Typical Diseases to which Indigo Ray subjects are prone: Eye troubles; Ear and Nose complaints; Facial Paralysis, etc.; also the following diseases may be remedied by use of Indigo: all diseases of the Lungs; Pneumonia, Bronchitis, Bronchial Croup; Whooping Cough; Asthma, Phthisis, Dyspepsia; nervous complaints such as Creeping Palsy; Infantile Convulsions; and also the Mental complaints: Delirium Tremens, Obsession, and other forms of Insanity.

Characteristics and effects of Indigo: This colour is a great purifier of the physical bloodstream, and also a tremendous mental freeing and purifying agent, controlling the psychic currents of our finer bodies. Indigo combines the deep Blue of Devotion and clear logical thought, with the faintest trace of the stabilizing Red tone. So it is a Ray combining great power and practicality; one upon which sweeping reforms take place at all levels of our being. Indigo is electric, cooling, and astringent; it induces local, and upon occasion total, anæsthesia.

Locality and Affinity: Indigo is related to the Frontal Chakram, situated behind the brow, anciently termed the Third Eye, controlling the Pineal Gland; it governs physical and higher vision, hearing, and olfaction. Indigo, in its effect on the mind, has an affinity with its complementary colour Yellow. Spiritually, Indigo is the Ray of the Holy Ghost vibration which indicates its great value in removing Obsession.

There are grounds for believing that Fear in the mind, *i.e.* shallow or perverted outlook, produces in the finals, the lung diseases above mentioned. This emotion sometimes centres around the navel brain centre, the seat of Dyspepsia, thereby stopping the natural currents, and hindering in the physical body the flow of digestive juices. Again the Fear that enters deeply into the psychic brain, bolstered by poisonous stimulants, shatters the aura and often results in Delirium Tremens, Obsession and the like. All need the purifying, stabilizing and immunizing rays of the Indigo vibration. Thus we may glimpse the tremendous importance of this agent in our world of to-day, in adjusting fears, frustrations, and the perversions of our inner energies.

Through evolving centuries, Man has extended his world of consciousness. He has, in general, risen out of the consciousness of an entirely physical world, and is already functioning widely in a constantly extending mental world. Through Science and Invention he has contacted basic laws and principles which have presented to his mind the inevitability of the existence of wider worlds still—Kingdoms of the Spirit. He stands at our time hesitant, uncertain, trying to place his feet safely on New Paths. Indigo, the Ray of New Race consciousness, is his stabilizer, his Light-bearer; it is the Ray promoting our deeper seeing and feeling into the true realities of Life, to make them clearer to our united understanding.

Since Indigo deals with the capacity to enlarge our comprehension, let us consider first those diseases which affect our organs of perception, the eyes, ears and nose.

Cataract: One such case treated with Indigo was that of a young woman who had built up a stony attitude towards her mother and step-father. Quite adamantly she had refused to see things their way and deeply resented rebuke or suggestion. She had gradually developed a persecution complex and her *outlook* on Life became warped. Cataract developed in the left eye.

Psychological treatment was first given to soften the unrelenting attitude and to relax her views. To this end the Universal breathing affirmation was suggested and she was given a wax rose of delicate salmon-pink colour to meditate upon. She was advised to increase this tint in her living quarters—she had told me that these were furnished mostly in dark brown.

In cases of this type, in order to relax the fixity of consciousness and then to raise the outlook, it is recommended to flood the treatment room with this soft pink light before treatment with the specific colour of the sight centre, until much of the harshness is dissolved from the mentality. Suggest the idea of breathing in this Peachy-Salmon radiation of goodwill to *All*.

In this instance, Indigo breathing was then commenced, and both eyes were bathed with Indigolo, and wet compresses of Indigolo were laid on the eyes and forehead, inducing complete relaxation. Dispensing with the second change of Indigolo compresses, the Indigolume was then focused on the eyes and forehead, with the request for deeper inhalation. Whilst light treatment continued for thirty minutes, the forehead was etherically massaged with the finger-tips. At this stage the healer, whilst affirming, may well visualize the Indigo power flowing through the finger-tips to the patient.

As this patient was unable to visit but once a week a transparent Indigo eyeshade was made, so that the patient could sit out in the sunshine in leisure moments and thus receive solarized Indigo rays directly on the eyes. The patient's outlook steadily improved with the softening influences and the stimulating Ihdigo treatment toned the eyes to their true vibration. The left eye cleared partially and became more vital. The completion of the cure was not witnessed as the patient was called away from the district.

Ivah B. Whitten, A.M.I.C.A., offers the case of a Miss X, who was distressed by the thought of encroaching blindness consequent upon a shock she had received. Medical examination proved there was no organic disease involved but that the psychological impress was affecting this centre of sensitivity. The point was reached where the patient could barely distinguish nearby objects. When the "Colour factor" was introduced to the treatment she was taken out of a Yellow and Orange Room and placed in a room of three shades of Green home-furnishings, with Violet light treatments twice each day. She was opposed to the study of Colour so her restoration was much slower. In seven weeks, however, the patient recovered part sight and could read large print, and in seven months acuity was almost normal.

Eva Longbottom, the blind musician-composer, in the appendix to her book "The Silver Bells of Memory" urges that the Blind Institute take up this most beautiful method of treatment with a deeper awareness of the underlying principles.

Deafness: This long-suffering complaint is sometimes caused through an accident or severe shock. Quite often, however, it is caused through an inverted mental or emotional attitude towards friends and relatives, by a refusal to be told anything, an unwillingness to hear certain things which may be good for one to hear.

In one family there were three middle-aged sisters; two had for many years been constantly upset by the machinations of the third, who kept up a continual emotional ferment between them. The two more passive sisters got tired and weary of hearing of the troubles made by the third and finally closed their ears, bottling up their emotions instead of transmuting them in forgiveness. The third sister persisted her vituperation. The two other sisters became deaf.

Such cases mentally shut their ears and give their subconsciousness the silent command, turning their auras inwards in self-centredness. In the wide view deafness is often caused by a shutting of the ears to the afflictions and affairs of the world, deaf to its pleas, a bottling up of attention within circumscribed self-interests, thus imposing limitations on the organism.

On the other hand, deafness is sometimes the result of over-willingness to hear and enlarge evil gossip, or again it may be the reaped result of some such cruelty sown in a former incarnation.

Treatment, in the first instance, should comprise an effort to release the self-centredness, to get them to entertain new ideas, until new suggestions are pleasantly awaited and even eagerly anticipated, until, in an attitude of ready approval they volunteer, "Hear! Hear!" A welcome affirmation. This release may often be aided through the Peachy-Pink light and affirmation.

Specific colour treatment starts with the patient gently breathing the Indigo Rays in affirmation, and bathing the face, and particularly the ears, with Indigolo as a start to each day. Then focus the Indigolume on the ear to be restored.

Ear-trumpets made of ugly brown tortoiseshell have often been observed, and it is submitted that such colours around a deaf patient but induce self-centredness. Celastoid and rhodoid of Indigo colour can be moulded into any desired shape nowadays, therefore the makers of these ear-funnels could work *with* treatment instead of against, if they substituted the colour stimulating the hearing centre. Indigo light might thus fall upon the defective drum. Those using the button device might have an outer-overlapping concave shell of clear Indigo celastoid that would *concentrate* Indigo light-waves into the ear drum.

Loss of Sense of Smell: Use the Universal Peachy-Pink breathing affirmation and imagine you are capable of inhaling the most delightful variety of flowers in the world. Place the suggestion in the mind of a wealth of awaiting beauty and fragrance.[1] Then sniff a little Indigolo up the nostrils two or three times a day, and gargle the back of the nose in the roof of the mouth. Using a piece of Indigo coloured silk, make a compress with Indigolo, unfold and spread it over the nose projecting Indigolume through it on to the etheric olfactory centres behind the nose. Inhale deeply through the nose to the Indigo breathing affirmation, particularly the lines:

"O Deep Rays of Indigo Blue,
Bring me in Devotion's hours,
New found fragrance in brain-flowers
Sweeping all brown leaves away."

To help capture the right mood, have a Vase of Altar Lilies nearby frequently, and project Indigolume through

---

[1] The Rishi Vishudhananda of Benares can demonstrate the separation of any perfume in the world you may desire out of the all-embracing Sun's rays by simple means of a small concentrating lens and his concentrated thought. If we Westerners who have vaunted the unfolding of the mind's powers outwardly could but concentrate our mental powers inwardly to ampli y our fulness of sight, hearing and olfaction, we should be able to remove many of our encasing limitations. In the Golden Age of Atlantis the advanced peoples had extended faculties of sight, hearing and olfaction extending great distances. We are also told that the bee was brought to this planet many thousands of years ago by the Lords of Flame, from Venus—a planet further evolved than the Earth. It is noteworthy that the bee also has powers of olfaction of many miles' range. Yet there are no powers inhering to the lesser Kingdoms of Life that are not also inhering to the Higher Kingdoms—of evolution, *e.g.* the Human stratum—we should realize that for the most part these faculties are merely latent.

them as you breathe in their elevating fragrance of devotion.

· · ·

Bleeding from the Nose: Snuffing, and bathing the nose in, Indigolo will stop the bleeding if it is caused by a rush of blood. Indigolume focused on the nose will prove greatly helpful also. If a person is accustomed to nose-bleeding, one dose of Indigolo at bed-time for a week will permanently stop the complaint.

Creeping Palsy: Ivah Bergh Whitten, A.M.I.C.A., contributes light on the treatment of this disease. It is primarily the result of mental helplessness or inability to control the individual expression.

"The patient must relax, mentally, and turn loose everything that has been worrying him, concentrating only upon the word SERENITY with all that the word implies, knowing that DIVINE MIND is all-powerful to rebuild every atom of the body and brain and to remove every adverse influence that may affect the harmony of life.

"Place him under the Blue light (Cerulume), passing it *down* the right side and *up* the left. Then starting with Deep Green (Verdilume) upon the soles of the feet, gradually move up until the spine is flooded with the Green. Then turn to Indigo (Indigolume) on the throat centre for twenty minutes. Afterwards proceed *down* the *right* side and *up* the *left*, pausing for ten minutes to concentrate the Indigo upon the soles of the feet.

"At night the patient should have a warm bath, of a temperature pleasing to the patient (but *not* cold), with the Indigo light over the tub and with Indigo cloths used to rub the body after the bath until the skin glows from the increase of circulation.

"If assistance cannot be given in the tub, bathe him in bed on a rubber sheet, with a warmed light blanket to protect him from cold. Use an Indigo salt-bag[1] in place of the sponge or wash-cloth, with the Indigo light shining over the bed.

"These salt-bags are made of doubled cheese-cloth and filled with two cupfuls of raw bran and half a cupful of common table salt. Then colour-charge the salt with Indigo, with the aid of the Sun or a lamp, for one hour.

"Should the patient not respond *at once* to the treatments

[1] Indigosal (see Table of Terminology for Colour-Solarized Substances, page 21).

let him have in addition the Indigo light over him as he sleeps, but reserve this extreme measure for emergency!"

Infantile Convulsions: Indigolume on the face and head soon soothes the young one and makes the condition serene.

Obsession: There are certain kinds of insanity that need deeper basic understanding than have been afforded them hitherto. Obsession is one of these. First of all, obsession of the bodily and mental vehicles of an individual is impossible where that individual's auric shell is intact, and where the egoic will is strong. A second, or foreign entity has the power to intrude only where there is sensitivity coupled with weak or surrendered will (mediumship), or where through some abuse of the creative centres, one or more, of the normally barred gateways (Chakra) into the protective aura have been broken down. The remedy is to re-orient the entity and to reseal the auric shield against possibility of violation.

One such case was that of a boy whose mother had been greatly attached to her brother before marriage. Evidently the brother had been a repressed type and keenly resentful of his sister's marriage, which he unsuccessfully tried to prevent. He died before the birth of his nephew. After puberty the boy was tempted to sexual abuse with the resultant breaking down of the auric shield, and obsession was accomplished by the "earth-bound" uncle who expressed many of his previously repressed ideas through the youngster.

Throughout the years of adolescence there were frequent periods of obsession during which the boy exhibited great precociousness and craftiness, indulging in the wildest escapades that frequently landed him in the hands of the police.

After years with ineffectual specialists, he came to Colour.

Upon the first treatment of the case the entity was contacted metaphysically and there was violent opposition and scorn until finally the effect of the Universal Love affirmation was felt by him. When it was impressed that we were working as much to help the entity reach his rightful sphere as we were to stabilize the boy, the former relectantly gave ground.

There followed a month or two during which the boy was free from obsession, and we obtained his co-operation to use opportunity to begin re-sealing the aura. This was done, to a considerable extent, by the use of Indigolume reinforced by the boy's egoic Ray vibration.

There followed a long period during which the boy was relatively free from obsession. I say relatively because two lapses occurred through the strength of former habits not yet completely eradicated, and which re-opened the breach in the aura causing a re-issued invitation to the entity.

Treatment was strengthened by a further fuller understanding with the boy and an Indigo lamp was permanently fixed above his bed so that he could switch it on at night when under duress. The lamp was very successfully used this way with only one further crisis when the entity urged cunningly that the boy smash the lamp to pieces. The youth resisted the temptation to acquiesce and thus won a firm step towards the final victory and freedom.

In repeating such treatment it would be well to bathe all orifices night and morning with Indigolo, and constantly to breathe deep in the Indigo vibration, raising the tone of consciousness in all ensuing activities. White is, of course, the Arch Ray for curing obsession, as it is for all disease. In the White of Christ Consciousness there can be no disease. Few can as yet reach up to use this Power Ray, but there is promise in the Rainbow, for through the gateways of colour we are led up to understand every component of the White. That is the purpose of Colour-Knowing.

Delirium Tremens has certain similarities with Obsession. In both instances there is a deterioration of the auric shield and impairment of the emotional, mental and astral vehicles through excess and abuse. The closing of the Astral door (through which they have contacted the monstrosities on the lower astral plane), and the regaining of the balanced faculties is obtained through Indigolume. Indigolo taken internally and regularly will help cleanse the system.

Exorcism: "Earth-bound" souls are liberated from their haunting delusions and attachments (causing them to re-enact their earthly lives or to prey on others), through Indigolume. Indigo again, is second only to the White Light in all forms of exorcism. Its vibrations are so powerful that all that is noble and worthy in the soul is stimulated, called-forth, uplifted and salvaged out of the dross of physical and lower-emotional consciousness. Moreover, real White is far too powerful to attempt to administer in the average case.

Anæsthesia: Indigolume is of unique value for inducing the safest and easiest form of anæsthesia known to science.

Though hardly appreciated or understood as yet, one or two manipulative surgeons, such as Dr. Kolar of Wichita, Kansas, are using it considerably for certain types of operations.

Under colour anæsthesia the patient is fully conscious yet oblivious of pain. This is because the Indigolume raises the consciousness to such a high rate of vibration that it becomes detached from awareness of happenings in the physical body. This is by no means colour-induced hypnosis, as some of the unaware have suggested. It is rather the withdrawing of the patient's consciousness to super-physical levels, yet *without any loss of identity-awareness*.

.   .   .

In all cases where there is inflammation it is best first to reduce heat by using straight Blue (Cerule), then to treat with Indigo to restore normal, or better, functioning. The following complaints come in this class.

Inflammation of the Eyes: This is caused either by diseases of the digestive organs, or by exposure, or by external injuries. When the cause is the digestive organs, light and cooling things should be taken and heating things avoided. Externally, Blue spectacles will help reduce the inflammation and then if Indigolume be thrown on the entire face, cure will be completed.

Granular Lids, Chronic Ulcerated Cornea: Often lancing of the inner sides of the lids is resorted to in the former disease, but if the above treatment is adhered to, total cure can be effected in a few weeks. Cerulume and Indigolume, as well as Indigolo, are also good for sore eyes, bloodshot eyes, and for stye.

Earache: Exposure sometimes causes a pimple or swelling in the ear with resulting inflammation. Cerulume will reduce the inflammation, and a Ceruleo syringe will cure the pimple with discharge from the ear. Care should always be taken that the cure is slow, otherwise sudden changes would deaden the ear and deafness follow. Complete cure and tonicity is obtained when finishing the treatment with Indigolume and Indigolo.

Abnormal Sounds in the ears are generally caused by an accumulation of heat in the brain. It can be cured by keeping the bowels open and the feet warm. Indigolume on the head will remove heat and normalize hearing.

Dyspepsia: Indigolume and Indigolo check the bad irritating humour, stop vomiting or purging and give a healthy tone to the digestive organs.

Dry Irritating Cough: This can be cured very easily by taking Indigolo. This water wets the phlegm so that it is thrown off sooner and without much effort; thus the patient feels relief.

Asthma: See section on the Orange Ray. When disease has not become chronic, Indigo will give relief in some cases. Such persons are generally those who have red colour predominant in their systems (Red Ray subjects) and who expose themselves to cold.

Mucous Fevers, Whooping Cough, Phthisis: All of these require Indigo treatment.

Pneumonia is another disease which shows an abnormal accumulation of heat in the lungs. Ceruleo would not be as beneficial as Indigolo since the lungs always require a little red (unless there is hæmorrhage, when Ceruleo remains best). As Indigo possesses this it acts like a charm on the lungs and reduces all heat, stops ulceration, checks the fever, and the patient is very soon cured, often within twenty-four hours.

Acute Bronchitis can be cured easily with Indigolo.

Insanity, Hallucinations, Delusions, Melancholia, Mania, Hypochondria, Senile Dementia, Hysteria, Epilepsy, Sexual Abuses, etc: It is advisable to use Indigo for the excitable cases and only Orange for those cases in which there is debility. Indigo, correctly applied, will thus do incalculable good.

Healing Colour-Breathing Affirmation
VIOLET RAY

O Zenith Ray of Violet Power
Cleanse my dark blood with Purple shower,
Soothe Thou my nerves when passions lower,
Bring forth true Inspiration's flower.

.   .   .

O Amethyst Ray of Spirit's radiance
Strike Thou the chord of my soul's cadence,
Bring forth the Poetry, Music, Fragrance,
One Art uniting—none in vagrancy.

.   .   .

O Violet blaze in meditation's bower
Flash me keen Intuition's power,
Dull mental shades no more shall dower
Thy Mystic, Petalled Lotus Flower.

.   .   .

The humble, modest Violet slight—
Shows Arrogance: "Power in Simple Might,"
Guides egos from dark paths of night,
In Service, Selfless, Endless Light.

Over the Desert at Sunset often spread veils of purest Amethyst, soothing out the day's harsh lights.

Presently, encroaching Dusk aeepens, to smoothest tones of Violet across the Wide expanse.

All the world is still with its magic. In utter quietude, it is yours. Silently take this gift from the Supreme Artist-Physician.

In joyous reverence breathe in its healing tonic to every nerve-fibre, its inspiration to every intuitive cell, to nourish and uplift All spiritual life within.

Chapter XI

VIOLET

METALS radiating Violet: Manganese, Barium, Aluminium, Iron, Rubidium, Calcium, Cobalt, Strontium, Titanium.

Chemicals: Silver Chloride, Arsenic, etc.

Best glass to use in the treatment of disease contains Manganese and Cobalt.

Foods: Aubergine, Purple Broccoli, Beet-tops; Purple Grapes, Blackberries, etc.

Typical diseases to which Violet Ray subjects are prone: Nervous and mental disorders; Neurosis, Neuralgia, Sciatica, and diseases of the scalp. Violet treatment will also remedy Epilepsy, Cerebro-Spinal Meningitis, Concussion, Cramps, Rheumatism, Tumours, Kidney and Bladder weaknesses. Violet animates and cleanses the venous blood.

Philosophy, Characteristics and effects of the Violet Ray: The Violet Rays are, of all others, those possessing the most intense electro-chemical power. Violet is acidulous. The extreme Violet-Purple Rays are very stimulating to the nervous system. The Trans-Violet, or Ultra-Violet Rays are not electrical but rather a higher grade of thermism, a grade so fine as to convey but a feeble, if any, impression of heat to the outward senses. Yet these higher grades of heat and cold can be felt by certain persons when in a specially sensitive condition. It is the ideal Purifier, and the purifier of ideals. Its high rate of frequency is depressing to the moronic mind because its potencies are beyond their understanding; it is stimulative mainly to the Intuitive (Spiritual) nature. Violet has great inspirational effect, e.g. the great works of Art, in Music, Prose, Poetry, Painting, Sculpture, etc., are indebted to the Violet Ray, the stimulator of highest human ideals.

Violet provides nourishment for all those cells in our upper brain that expand the horizon of our Divine Understanding. Leonardo da Vinci, the famous painter and one of the greatest investigators of the Science of Colour, maintained that our power of meditation can be increased tenfold if we meditate under the rays of the Violet light falling softly through the stained-glass windows of a quiet church. Wagner had violet draperies and materials about him when composing or bringing through, music of the highest spiritual quality. The famous Comte de St. Germain used the purifying violet rays to heal the sick and to remove the clouds and blemishes from gems. All these instances illustrate the spiritual impetus which the high frequencies of Violet impart.

A well-known English clergyman says that he believes one of the results of our nervous dissatisfaction with our world comes from the realization of failure in our religious life—the lack of that poise which comes with Inner Knowing. Meditation in Amethyst advances this self-realization.

Locality and Affinity: Violet controls the Crown Chakram (known in the East as the Thousand-Petalled Lotus) and is linked in our physical bodies to the Pituitary Gland, that Intuitive Centre of spiritual perception, the counterpart of the Pineal Gland, or Third Eye. Violet, or Purple, is often termed the "Power Ray" which explains its association with kings—"Royal Purple". Just as a king is the all-powerful ruler over the body of his kingdom, so Purple, occupying the Throne Centre, crowns the Higher Mind, the ruler of the kingdom of the body, in all its component members, citadel-centres, organs of industry, and the billions of cell-subjects composing the nerves and tissues.

The Violet Ray is in two parts; the Amethyst, or spiritual part, and the Purple, or more temporal part more closely related to the earth plane.

This Purple half of the Ray is the colour reflex of the lust for power, deep, passionate, and ruthless. Through this self-assertive Red aspect, creeping into the Violet, unprepared, unevolved egos are led into spiritual degeneration.

Amongst those who have prepared themselves aright to deal with the coming of the Purple are the tranquil ones, who have transmuted it towards the Amethyst of balance and spirituality, and they have become great teachers and reformers, the promoters of mighty efforts of peace and service.

There is the classic example of the offer of the Purple of power in the Biblical story of the Temptation of Jesus when offered all the kingdoms of the world. But He chose the spiritualized Amethyst part of the Ray and He became a King in the things of the Spirit, rather than in the things of the Earth. To the world that choice might seem a failure and a confession of weakness; how wise that choice really was we may not realize until we more fully appreciate the Power of the Spirit. The key-note of the Violet-Amethyst Ray is Service, Selfless—even self-sacrificing, Service. Let us then consider how this Ray serves Man.

When the human system has a predominance of nervous and vascular excitement, Violet has a remarkable affinity for such conditions, bringing about harmony and health, as will be seen in the cases of neurosis, nervous irritation, neuralgia and inflammatory diseases of the nerves.

Neurosis has a supreme curative agent in Violet. This complaint is often found in active, high-strung types who just "live on their nerves". It predominates perhaps among creative artists such as musicians, actors, and singers, in which professions a great deal of nervous energy is used up. Such people are often keenly intuitive and lose themselves in the artistic and rapturous subtleties of other and finer worlds. But coming back to physical routine—details, necessities, problems and decisions—is a shock to their systems. The contrast is too extreme, too sudden, too noisy and jarring, and the wear and tear on the nerves is thus aggravated. The result is emotional opposition, or what is known as "temperamental tantrums", and injured pride. Amongst these we find also the Jekylls-and-Hydes, those suffering from Schizophrenia, or split personalities.

It is remarkable that many such artistes, in the depths of depressions, resort to drugs of the phosphorus base, this being a substance on the Yellow Ray[1] (a food for the nerves and intellectual brain), and complementary to the Violet Ray which nourishes the intuitive counterpart of the brain. They would do better if they took the stimulus in Yellow light-waves and avoided the injury of drugs. Where there is depression Yellow is invaluable for many; where there is irritation and excitability, Violet should be used always to poise and stabilise expression. Ambero and Purpuro respectively are easy forms of taking these tonics.

The Violet Breathing Affirmation is of great benefit practised in the early morning and at all times of stress. Purpurgas and Violume absorbed for half an hour morning and evening will serve to tone and regulate the nerves for a serene day's work, and to restore them for relaxing sleep at night.

[1] The spectrum of Phosphorus combines Yellow and Violet.

Concussion: A great friend of the author once suffered severe concussion as a result of the car, in which he was a passenger, being driven recklessly over a road ramp. His head hit a cross-frame in the roof of the machine, and for long weeks thereafter he could remember nothing. When finally allowed out alone he would often collapse in the street. For many months he remained half-bereft of his faculties and was incapable of turning back to the work in which he had been formerly engrossed.

Fortunately, his wife, a lady of deep understanding who had herself been cured from an "incurable" illness by Colour, persuaded him to acquiesce to colour treatment that was keyed to Violume. At once recovery began to be noticed and at the end of three months the improvement was remarkable. Soon afterwards he was putting forward new ideas in his work, and recently he took up important government assignments with the zest and eagerness that assured success.

Insomnia: The relaxing shades of Violet, Indigo and Blue are all specifics for sleeplessness, the ray and the shade depending upon the person. With the wide-spread increase of this disease the Blue-Amethyst range should be far more extensively employed.

Violet should rarely be used where there is lack of desire to express, or put forth, the creative ability, for with most people and particularly with morons, it acts as a deterrent or repressive agent, and the subject feels as a result "bottled up" and explosive. Yellow or Orange would add intelligent stimulus to self-expression, and Green would promote active application. Amethyst would *later* raise the expression to selfless endeavour—*Ars pro Artis*.

Dr. Edwin Babbitt gives an interesting case of Nervous Irritability in which he employed the ingredients of Violet, and which it might be helpful to quote:

"Mr. T., aged 35. In consequence of long continued excessive physical and mental exertion, his nervous system was entirely disordered; the derangement manifested itself in nervousness, and trying irritability; he could not sleep at night, was disturbed by frightful dreams; his appetite was variable, sometimes ravenous, at others, the very sight of food was an annoyance; his bowels varied too, at times constipated, at others lax; he had frequent pains in the head, the least excitement unnerved him, and he was inclined to extreme despondency. His irritability forbade Red light (Rubilume) so Blue (Cerulume) was administered with Rubigo internally. The beneficial results were immediate; his entire system improved rapidly; five treatments in all actually restored a healthy tone to his nervous system, and he has since experienced nothing of 'nervousness' though his life is one of constant physical and mental activity."

It will be noted that this treatment combined Blue and Red—resulting in Violet.

Neuralgic Headache: A city merchant came home from church one Sunday morning with a severe neuralgic head-ache, and although he had no special faith in colour, con-cluded he would try it. By sitting under Mazarine Blue-Violet glass for thirty minutes he was entirely relieved.

Colour for Lunacy: Over fifty years ago, Dr. Ponza, director of the lunatic asylum at Alessandria (Piedmont, Italy), having conceived the idea that the solar rays might have some curative power in diseases of the brain, communi-cated his views to Father Secchi of Rome, who replied: "The idea of studying the disturbed state of lunatics in connection with magnetic perturbations, and with the coloured, especially violet light of the sun, is of remarkable import-ance." Dr. Ponza, following the instructions of the learned Jesuit, prepared several rooms oriented to the East and South, each in a different colour supplied by the walls and windows, and several patients were kept there under observa-tion. One of them affected with morbid taciturnity became gay and affable after three hours in a Red chamber; another, a maniac who refused all food, asked for some breakfast after twenty-four hours in the same Red chamber. A highly excitable case in a strait-jacket was kept all day in a Blue chamber, and after but an hour he appeared much calmer. Another patient passed the night in a Violet chamber, and on the following morning begged Dr. Ponza to send him home because he felt himself cured, and he has remained so ever since. The principles of Colour are now used in many mental homes throughout the world.

Cramp: Adolphe von Gerhardt charged sugar of milk with Blue and Violet light and called it od[1] magnetic sugar

---

[1] "Od" is a term given by Dr. von Reichenbach of Vienna to the higher octave of Colour Vibrations.

(Cerulelac and Violac). He speaks of a babe near Jena, that was declared by its physicians to be "hopelessly lost" from having had a terrible series of cramps for four hours. He "poured a blade's endful of it into its mouth." In fifteen minutes the cramps ceased and the child soon became perfectly well.

Sciatica: "A remarkably vigorous and muscular young man of twenty-two years of age was afflicted with a severe attack of sciatica, or rheumatism of the sciatic nerve, in his left hip and thigh, for which he had been unable to obtain any relief, although the usual medical as well as galvanic remedies had been applied. He became almost lame from it and he suffered much pain in his attempts to walk. He was advised to try the associated Sun and Violet light, both upon his naked spine and hip. He did this with such benefit that at the end of three weeks after taking the first of these colour treatments, every symptom of the disorder disappeared and he has had no return of it since, a period of now three years."
—*Gen. Pleasanton.*

Spinal Meningitis requires treatment by Violet or Green all the way to the hips; Green being suitable for the lower spine. General Pleasanton relates an agreeable incident of a lady whose "daughter had four years since been afflicted with a violent attack of spinal meningitis. Her sufferings were indescribable but continuous. Every conceivable remedy had been resorted to during those four years, but without benefit. Her nervous system became at last so disordered that the slightest sound or the most gentle agitation of the air thre her into most agonizing suffering. She was wasted away in flesh, could not sleep at night, had no appetite, and her life was despaired of. The physician was dismissed and the young lady relied entirely upon Indigo-Violet colour treatment for her restoration to health. The lady said that on entering the room thus lighted, the pains from which she was suffering almost immediately ceased. They would return in a modified form on leaving the room, but grew less from day to day. Very soon her condition began to improve, her appetite returned, and with it her strength; she began to gain flesh, her sleeplessness disappeared, and in short, she was speedily restored to health."

Baldness: "A singular feature of the aforementioned case was that her hair all came out and she became quite bald.

Her physician examined the scalp with a microscope and declared there were no roots of hair remaining, and that consequently she would never again have a natural head of hair. This announcement to the young lady was worse than would have been a death-warrant," says the General. Under the Indigo-Violet treatment, however, the hair did begin to grow, the lady discarded her wig, and when called upon by General Pleasanton she showed him a luxuriant growth of hair which any young lady might envy.

Dandruff and Scurvy: Purpuro is good for these complaints alternated with Ceruleo. It is excellent for any diseases of the scalp.

Amaurosis and Cataract: Violet (as well as Indigo) is recommended for curing both these complaints, in the former Rubilume is also needed and "it is very important", says Dr. Babbitt, "to take Colour baths and massage to tone up the system."

Involuntary Discharge of Water: Purpurlume or Verdilume on the bladder will remove the weakness and make the neck of the organ more elastic at will, and the involuntary discharge will thus be stopped. It is, of course, advisable to withhold liquids at night.

Leucorrhea: Purpuro is considered better than Ceruleo for this female complaint.

Violet quickens the germination of higher forms of life in every kingdom. As we have seen in the foregoing, Violet is the subtlest refinement of Light and is the subtlest refiner of our finer bodies. Is it not an interesting comparison, by way of corollary and conclusion, to note that Violet light greatly facilitates the hatching of silkworms, the producers, until the advent of recent substitutes, of our finest medium for sheer light-transmitting-fabrics?

HEALING COLOUR-BREATHING AFFIRMATION
WHITE RAY

O Dazzling White, Pure Ray Serene—
Uplift my Soul to meet Thy Gleam;
Fill every Atom with Power Supreme,
Make Ill-thought Life seem but a dream.

.   .   .

O Resplendent Father, Seven Rays in One—
Teach me to blaze my Hidden Sun;
To Repent, Rejoice like Prodigal Son—
Homeward, with Seven-fold Life begun.

.   .   .

O Mighty Ray, Omniscient Power—
Thy Rainbow holds Heaven-scent of Man and Flou er;
The Cosmic Music blends in Thee
In Fragrant Radiant Symphony.

.   .   .

O Arch Transmuter-Protector, free
All limiting talents now boundlessly—
Love merged with Strength, no more diverse,—
Encompass the Vast of Universe!

Quiten every restless thought and expand into profound calm. Breathe deeply. Lift all the power-energy at your command to the very zenith-peak of your consciousness until all that is of white within you flashes forth to meet the first glimmer of Divine White descending.

Breathe deeply and multiply this White Light.—Surround yourself in its Protective Power. Then place the friend whom you wish to heal in its midst. Afterwards share it with all the sick in the world.

Chapter XII

WHITE

THERE are the potentialities of White in all metals, chemicals and all other substances. Although Platinum and Silver have been ascribed to the "White Ray", it is really the sole perquisite of none, but rather the ultimate of all. White is truly the Arch Transmuter of Metals and of Men—a manifestation of the Father Principle in the Universe—the All-Embracing.

The best Glass or Lenses to use in Treatment of disease should be made from Quartz, which transmits all the spectrum values of White sunlight.

Characteristics and Effects of White: The White Ray is not a Ray in the sense of the Colour Rays with which we have been dealing: it is a symposium of All Seven Rays—a perfect blending of the spectrum reproducing the original White light. White has the attribute of lifting and dynamizing any single Ray Colour and of transmuting that Ray to the peak of its characteristic potentialities.

Thus, White may be compared to the Electricity flowing into a Coloured bulb, which gains increasing dazzling luminosity as higher voltages are passed through it, thereby affording greater powers of human perception, making objects in the environment clearer. Similarly, the Cosmic White Light flowing into the bulb of consciousness, coloured with our particular Ray outlook, raises and expands our auric light, extending our powers of perception of inner and Cosmic realities.

Spiritually, The White Light is the Divine Radiance of The Father of the Cosmos—the Logos. It is the Light of Christ-Consciousness, of Supreme Power, Purity, Perfection —the Primary Healing Power. It is the Light of At-One-Ment with the Source of Life.

There is a radiant relationship between the spiritual Son of God (The Christ) and the so-called physical Sun of our zodiacal system. Just as the Divine Son was (and is) a focal centre of God's Life-Intelligence, so also the Sun is one of the dynamic focal centres of Divine Energy. The fact that our Sun and its solar system is only one amongst scores of other suns and solar systems larger than our own, does not lessen this beautiful relationship. After all, each individual has the Son of God spark within his own microcosmic system, a replica of the outer macrocosmic system, and there are many millions of souls and therefore many millions of micro-universes.

When, at the zenith of Human Consciousness, we perceive the reflection of the Divine Cosmic Light in our souls we experience a falling away of all that is dross, a transmutation of all our baser earthly elements of disease. This realization is achieved only by completely identifying ourselves with the Pure White Light of the Christ-Consciousness, whereby all negative conditions are wiped from our consciousness, and therefore from our lower bodies also. All shadows of disease dissolve as all bodily cells are purified with the White Flame of dazzling power.

Even so, at such great moments in our lives, we are permitted to receive but a greatly diminished, or transformed, potentiality of the Great White Ray. Its full dynamic force would utterly shatter the atomic structure of our bodies at our present stage of evolution. Nevertheless, the glimmer or reflection of this Dynamic Ray vouchsafed to us appears of the most tremendous dazzling power that we could possibly conceive or comprehend.

When healing with the Colour Rays (specialized from the White light) we are able to use one separated Ray specifically with understanding of its unique characteristics. As we gain healing knowledge of all the Seven Rays in diversity, we can appreciate more fully the wondrous summation unity affords us in all-round understanding of what White truly comprises. Colour therefore offers us the sevenfold path to comprehending the essential glory of the Divine Cosmic White Radiance, and it is through understanding and realization alone that we grow.

Often when a long-patient soul is ready to take the next step forward in evolution it receives a baptism or initiation with the White Ray, the seeds of disease in the consciousness are burnt up, limitations are dissolved and the awareness purified and expanded with wider vista of possibilities unfolded to view. Inevitably this comes as the climax, or earned reward to the faithful ones who have steadily plodded through the dark night pre-dawn consciousness of disease and suffering.

Under this All-Embracing Ray of Christ-Consciousness takes place all Healing through Faith such as witnessed at Lourdes and at Milton Abbey, whereafter in the healed soul there dwells a larger realization of the essential beauty of God's world for Man.

The White light, from higher planes, is truly a Divine Manna capable of vitalizing every living thing. It may be used to charge water by an effort of will power.

Those who are familiar with the remarkable healing work of the kindly Cagliostro, that great pupil of St. Germain, will recall that he healed many thousands of the poor and destitute of Paris without any apparent diagnosis—he just gave each one a little colourless liquid to drink. His success so astonished the physicians of his day, who, foreseeing the prospect of their practices vanishing, secretly obtained a sample of this liquid from one of Cagliostro's patients. It was analysed and pronounced to be merely water, and Cagliostro was denounced as a charlatan. However, his cures remained to honour him. It may be said that these were faith cures, but this explanation would hardly fit the majority of the cases. These were not miracles of healing, they were the benign outworking of the principles of pranic impregnation operated by one willing to work with nature's laws and forces instead of against them—the usual human habit.

Thus we see all Life empowered by the impetus of the Cosmic White Light.

Various eminent physicians, and researchers from the scientific rather than the theosophic view offer the following interesting facts reflecting on White.

Dr. Babbitt says: "Light, being an actual substance with peculiar styles of vibrations according to the particular colours which compose it, and at a rate of nearly 186,000 miles a second, it is easy to see that it must have great power, and that the substance receiving it must partake of this power. The fact that the whole world, mineral, vegetable, and animal, is ever being transformed into new and beautiful growths, forms and colours under its magic touch, shows its almost omnific power."

Reichenbach proved by many experiments upon persons of very delicate sensibilities, whom he called sensitives, the great and peculiar power of White sunlight. He had water stand in the sunlight for five minutes when Miss M., on drinking it without knowing what was done, said immediately that it was magnetized. "It produced a peculiarly pepper-like burning on her tongue, palate, throat, down to the stomach, at every point arousing symptoms." Water which stood twenty minutes in the sunshine was found to be as strongly magnetic as when charged with a nine-layered magnet.

"I allowed Miss R. to become used to feeling of my hand," says Reichenbach, "and then went out into the sunshine. After ten minutes had elapsed, during which time I had exposed myself on all sides to the sun's rays, I went back and gave her the same hand. She was so much astonished at the rapid alteration in the great increase of force which she experienced in it, the cause of which was unknown to her."

Sun Force can be bottled up in water as the following experiment by J. F. Waters, M.D., clearly shows: "I put a bottle of water in the sun for two days in a clear (transparent) bottle, then drank a couple of swallows, and for two days I thought it would burn me up. I could not believe it was the water, so after it was over, I repeated it with a smaller dose, and the effect was the same in proportion to the dose."

There are persons in delicate health so sensitive that they cannot drink ordinary water unless some magnetic person has held the ends of his fingers near it to charge it. If unmagnetized water is handed to them to drink, they will discover it at once and throw it aside with disgust. If such persons should sun-charge water it would doubtless become so magnetic as to answer every purpose. In fact all persons would receive a vitalizing power by drinking simply suncharged (or sun-kissed) water.

The toughening power of the sun was well illustrated by a lady patient of Dr. Babbitt. She was very feeble and negative, and every little exposure would cause her to take cold. She took a course of sun-baths on the skin over the lungs and other parts of her body, since when she rarely ever takes cold. In this respect she has become permanently strong, as years have elapsed without a recurrence of her old conditions.

Augustus Barnes remarks that he has studied the hygienic properties of light for many years: "I can remove cancers in their earlier stages, tumours, nevus maternus (or mother's marks). It matters not whether the latter are red, black, purple, brown or any other colour, or whether they cover the entire side of the face, or large protuberances appear, I remove all by a lens and the simple rays of the Sun, without starting a drop of blood or leaving a scar but a short time. There is less pain attending this operation than by common surgery. Uncomely moles that disfigure the faces of many persons can be made to disappear and leave the face as fair as nature intended it, nor do they ever reappear. This treatment produces no ill-effects, for there are no chemical or mineral poisons in the balanced rays of the Sun."

Advantages of the Sun's Rays over all other caustics and the lancet may be enumerated as follows:

1. There is no mutilation of any part, nor is a drop of blood ever drawn. The Sun's rays will cauterize a vein or an artery so as almost instantly to stop its bleeding.

2. There is no after dressing needed, except with cancers.

3. There are no bad after-effects resulting from poisoning, as with drugs, for the Sun's rays are not poisonous.

4. There is no scar left after a sufficient time has elapsed for the healing process; the redness caused will gradually disappear.

5. There is no loss of consciousness under operation.

6. Those who have been subjected to both systems express themselves as feeling less than half the pain under the Sun's rays.

7. Colour Anæsthetics serve to remove pain completely; drugs or gaseous anæsthetics are not required at all.

8. No detention from business, etc., is required.

9. The quickness and permanence of the treatment and the simplicity of the operation are remarkable. It is easily controlled, and the operator can burn to a considerable depth, or so slightly as to destroy only the cuticle, stopping the cauterization at any stage he pleases.

10. The remedy is to be found wherever the Sun shines, requiring no preparation, no grinding, no mixing; but is ready every day free to all.

The International Congress of Physicians meeting in Italy at the beginning of the present century declared that sunlight is the most practical of all antiseptics.

Pasteur demonstrated that rooms which admit no sunlight become over-charged with bacteria, and everyone is aware of the fact that close rooms have a lifeless smell.

Dr. Forbes Winslow, in his volume "Light, and its influence on Life and Health", says: "The total exclusion of the sunbeams induces the severer forms of chlorosis, green sickness, and other anæmic conditions depending upon an impoverished and disordered state of the blood. Under these circumstances the face assumes a death-like paleness, the membranes of the eyes bloodless, and the skin shrunken and turned to a waxen colour; also emaciation, muscular debility and degeneration, dropsical effusion, softening of the bones, general nervous excitability, morbid irritability of the heart, loss of appetite, tendency to syncope and hæmorrhages, consumption, physical deformity, stunted growth, mental impairment and premature old age."

Dr. Ellsworth says: "Shut from sunlight, tubercles are formed in the lungs. The popular snow frolicking treatment for tubercular children, is beneficial not only because of the purity and dryness of the air in mountain altitudes, the temperature inducing toughness of fibre, but because the snow, reflecting all the light rays in total white, concentrates to heal all conditions."

"Who has not observed the purifying effect of Light," says the revered Florence Nightingale, "and especially the direct Sunlight; the usefulness of light in treating disease is all-important. Where there is Sun, there is thought, all physiology goes to confirm this. Put the sickly plant or human being into the sunshine, and if not too far gone, each will recover health and strength."—"Notes on Nursing."

Paul Brunton, in his valuable book, "A Search in Secret India", relates how the Rishi Vishudhananda of Benares will pick up a bird that has fallen lifeless to the ground and hold it in the warmth of his hands. Then holding an ordinary pocket concentrating lens he will focus the Sun's rays into the eyes of the bird, and it will flutter to life and fly about for half an hour, then die again. Undoubtedly the sun-power has a great charging influence upon the life-forces and fluids.

"It is a well established fact," says Dr. Forbes Winslow, "that as the effect of isolation from the stimulus of light, the fibrine, albumen and red-blood-cells become diminished in quantity, and the serum or watery portion of the vital fluid, augmented in volume, thus inducing a disease known to physicians and pathologists as Leukæmia—an affection in which the white instead of the red blood-cells are developed.

This exclusion from the Sun produces the sick, flabby, pale, anæmic condition of the face, or ex-sanguined ghostlike forms so often seen amongst those not freely exposed to air and light."

Such are the facts regarding the White Ray, deduced from experiment, experience, research, realization and living-philosophy. It remains with the student to regard the beacon sign-posts planted by others, and in their light to experience for himself, choosing the method of applying his knowledge that best suits his inner inclinations, until the time arrives when, perhaps, he may prove readily eager to use them in their totality.

BIBLIOGRAPHY

WHAT COLOUR MEANS TO YOU. By Ivah Bergh Whitten, A.M.I.C.A. (Daniel).

COLOUR BREATHING: The Breath of Transmutation. By Ivah B. Whitten, A.M.I.C.A. (Daniel).

THE LIGHT OF IVAH B. WHITTEN. By D. A. Bailey (A.M.I.C.A.).

LESSONS IN COLOUR AWARENESS. By Ivah Bergh Whitten (a correspondence course, issued by A.M.I.C.A., Calif.).

COLOUR AND CANCER. By C. E. Iredell, M.D.(London), M.R.C.P. (H. K. Lewis).

THE WISDOM OF THE SPIRIT. By Armido (A.M.I.C.A., Calif.).

HEALING IN THE LIGHT OF THE WISDOM OF THE SPIRIT. By Armido (A.M.I.C.A., Calif.).

THE PRINCIPLES OF LIGHT AND COLOUR. By Edwin D. Babbitt, M.D., LL.D.

RESEARCHES ON LIGHT AND ITS CHEMICAL RELATIONS. By Professor Robert Hunt, F.R.S.

CHROMOPATHY. By Jwala Prasada, F.T.S., Munsiff of Benares.

SPIRITUAL CHROMATICS. By John Hyde Taylor.

COLOUR AND YOU. By René Edouin (Dr. Hylton).

THE INFLUENCE OF COLOUR ON OUR MIND AND HEALTH. By Oscar Brunler (Uma Press).

A TREATISE ON THE SEVEN RAYS. By Alice A. Bailey (Lucis Press, in 5 Vols.).

THE NEW SCIENCE OF COLOUR. By Beatrice Irwin (Rider).

THE GATES OF LIGHT. By Beatrice Irwin (Rider).

THE FIFTH DIMENSION. By Vera Stanley Alder (Rider).

THE INITIATION OF THE WORLD. By Vera Stanley Alder (Rider).

The Finding of the Third Eye. By Vera Stanley Alder (Rider).

Fragrant and Radiant Healing Symphony, Colour, Sound, Perfume. By Roland Hunt, A.M.I.C.A., (Daniel).

The Science of Seership. By Geoffrey Hodson (T. S. Publishing House).

The Coming of the Angels. By Geoffrey Hodson (T. S. Publishing House).

New Light on The Treatment of Disease. By Geoffrey Hodson (T. S. Publishing House).

Colour in Health and Disease. By C. G. Sanders, F.R.C.P., D.Sc. (Daniel).

Spectro-Biology. By Maryla de Chrapowicki (Daniel).

The Laws of Operation. By Ebba G. Keenan (Daniel).

Cosmos, Man and Society. By Edmond Székely (Daniel).

The Salts of Salvation. By Eudora Perry and Dr. Carey.

The World Breath. By L. C. Beckett (Rider).

Some Unrecognised Factors in Medicine. By The T. S. Research Centre (T. S. Publishing House).

A Search in Secret India. By Paul Brunton (Rider).

Psychic Healing. By Ramacharaka. (Fowler).

The Technique of The Master. By Raymund Andrea (A.M.O.R.C., Calif.).

Co-operative Healing. By L. E. Eeman (Daniel).

Unseen Servers. By Dorothy A. Bailey.

Watchers of The Seven Spheres. By H. K. Challoner. (Routledge).

The Harmony of The Spheres. By Margery Livingston (Wright & Brown).

Signposts to Colour Healing. By H. M. Whitehead.

INDEX

(Compiled by the kindness of Miss E. M. Fletcher, A.M.I.C.A.)

123